Planning and Evaluating Health Programs:
A Primer

To: Dilna, Dianne, and Judy

Planning and Evaluating Health Programs: A Primer

Charles D. Hale, Ed.D., C.H.E.S.
Frank Arnold, D.P.A.
Marvin T. Travis, D.P.A.

Delmar Publishers Inc.

I(T)P™

NOTICE TO THE READER

Delmar Staff

Senior Acquisitions Editor: William Burgower
Senior Administrative Assistant: Debra Flis
Project Editor: Carol Micheli
Production Coordinator: Mary Ellen Black
Art and Design Manager: Russell Schneck
Design Coordinator: Karen Kemp

For information, address Delmar Publishers Inc.
3 Columbia Circle, Box 15-015
Albany, New York 12212

Copyright © 1994
by Delmar Publishers Inc.
The trademark ITP is used under license.

printed in the United States of America
published simultaneously in Canada
by Nelson Canada,
a division of The Thomson Corporation

4   5   6   7   8   9   10   XXX   00   01

Library of Congress Cataloging-in-Publication Data

Hale, Charles D., 1954–
    Planning and evaluating health programs : a primer / by Charles D.
Hale, Frank Arnold, Marvin T. Travis.
        p.   cm.
    Includes index.
    ISBN 0-8273-5448-7
    1. Health planning—Methodology.   2. Health planning.   3. Public
health—Evaluation.   4. Management information systems.   I. Arnold,
Frank, 1939–   .   II. Travis, Marvin T.   III. Title.
RA394.H35   1994
362.1'0684—dc20   92-47070
                                                              CIP

Contents

Preface

Experience in community and public health has convinced the authors of the need for this book. This observation has been confirmed by conversations with fellow public health practitioners and others practicing within the various health disciplines over the years.

After conferring with colleagues, both within and without the classroom, this volume was developed and is now offered. It is our hope that it will be of some use to those who labor in the hope of protecting and nurturing the public's health.

Following is a brief description of the present works purpose, intended audience, assumptions, and instructional objectives, as well as an overview of each of its chapters. Each example has been carefully developed to reinforce points made in the text.

PURPOSE, AUDIENCE, AND ASSUMPTIONS

The purpose of this work is to assist operations health program managers to more efficiently and effectively plan, manage, and evaluate their programs. The authors have emphasized an applied approach to this presentation.

Three models are presented: (a) an operations health program planning model, (b) a program evaluation model, and (c) a planning documentation model. When combined, these three models provide a comprehensive, integrated health program planning and evaluation model. Presented in subsequent chapters are supporting discussions concerning demography, epidemiology, health services research, budgeting, implementation strategies, and management information systems as related to operations health planning.

A detailed discussion of planning history, planning theory, and strategic planning are beyond the scope of this work. Additionally, it has been assumed by the authors that those using this book have a functional understanding of their health specialty.

INSTRUCTIONAL OBJECTIVES

This volume is divided into three sections which are designed to be instructive to the reader. Section IV consists of two contributed cases for the reader to review. In the next few paragraphs, outlined are instructional objectives which should be achievable once the relevant section of the book has been read and carefully studied.

After carefully studying Section I (Operations Health Planning and Evaluation), the reader will be able to (a) describe the strategic management process, (b) describe and employ the operational health planning model, (c) describe and use the program evaluation model, and (d) utilize the health planning documentation model. Instructional objectives are related to the following chapters:

Objective Ia	Chapter 1
Objective Ib	Chapter 2
Objective Ic	Chapter 3
Objective Id	Chapter 4

Upon careful study of Section II (Health Planning Methods), the reader will be able to (a) describe, read, and interpret the types of data [demographic, epidemiological, and health services research] commonly utilized in health planning; (b) apply descriptive statistics to demographic and epidemiologic data; (c) summarize descriptive data into tables, charts, and graphs; (d) describe the survey research process as well as a recommended format for reporting results; (e) construct a line item budget; and (f) describe and employ three program implementation strategies. Instructional objectives are related to the following chapters:

Objective IIa	Chapters 5, 6, & 7
Objective IIb	Chapters 5, 6, & 7
Objective IIc	Chapter 6
Objective IId	Chapter 7
Objective IIe	Chapter 8
Objective IIf	Chapter 9

After careful study of Section III (Management Information Systems), the reader will be able to (a) describe the computer in terms of its parts, types, capabilities, and limitations; (b) describe the recommended relationship between the computer user and an organization's information services department; (c) describe commonly applied computer security techniques; (d) describe four MIS applications; and (e) describe the relationship between MIS and health planning. Instructional objectives are related to the following chapters:

Objective IIIa	Chapter 10
Objective IIIb	Chapter 10
Objective IIIc	Chapter 10
Objective IIId	Chapter 11
Objective IIIe	Chapter 11

All chapters (except chapter 4) have review and/or application questions presented at the end of the chapter. Answers to these 163 questions are presented after the two cases. Also, thirty-five discussion questions are included.

BRIEF OVERVIEW OF CHAPTERS

In the next few pages, the general contents of each chapter is presented. Within each chapter are referrals to more detailed, specialized books on each topic.

Presented within chapter 1 (The Planning Challenge) are general comments concerning health planning and a discussion of strategic management.

Chapter 2 (An Operations Health Planning Model) contains the following: (a) an introduction to an operations health planning model, (b) definition of key planning terms, (c) a classification scheme for program objectives, (d) a presentation of an integrated operational health planning model, (e) the Hardee Cog Company Case, and (f) construction of a Gantt Chart.

Discussed in chapter 3 (A Program Evaluation Model) are: an overview of evaluation, types and purpose of evaluation studies, an operations level program evaluation model, and the Hardee Cog Company Case. Selected issues in evaluation are discussed.

Outlined in chapter 4 (A Planning Documentation Model) is a model for preparing an operations oriented health planning document with a discussion of the contents of each section. An example, The Hardee Cog Company, is presented.

Presented in chapter 5 (Health Planning Methods: Demography) is an analytical framework for interpreting demographic data and a discussion of the descriptive application of demography to operations health planning.

Within chapter 6 (Health Planning Methods: Epidemiology), a discussion of epidemiologic data, various descriptive indices (rates, ratios, proportions, and measures of central tendency) are explained and uses profiled. Additionally, guidelines for constructing tables, charts, and graphs are presented along with examples.

In chapter 7 (Health Planning Methods: Health Services Research), a discussion of descriptive health services research (HSR), descriptive HSR indices and applications, the survey research process, and HSR design considerations is presented. Sampling, data collection methods (questionnaire, interview, and document review) are discussed.

In chapter 8 (Health Planning Methods: Budgeting), discussed are the line-item and program budgets; models for constructing specific line items (staffing, travel, office support, educational materials, clinical materials, continuing education, and other costs); and preparing budget justification statements.

Presented in chapter 9 (Health Planning Methods: Implementation Strategies), are three strategies to ease plan implementation: organization development, negotiation, and marketing.

In chapter 10 (Management Information Systems: Introduction) is a discussion of the development of a computer based information system, types of computers, computer capabilities and limitations, security, and purchase decisions.

Presented in chapter 11 (Management Information Systems: Applications) is a discussion of traditional and modern MIS applications. Modern MIS applications include local area networks, decision support systems, expert systems, electronic data interchange, and interorganizational data interchange.

CDH
FA
MTT

Acknowledgments

We would like to thank Ms. Clarissa Simmens, Mrs. Cindy Plemons, Ms. Valerie Studnick, and Dr. Dilna M. Hale for editing and proofing the present work.

Thanks go to Dr. Steve Dorman (University of Florida), Dr. Mary Sutherland (Florida State University), and Ms. Kelly Shaw (Washington State Government) for their comments and suggestions.

CDH
FA
MTT

About the Authors

Charles D. Hale, Assistant Professor of Health Care Administration, joined the Saint Leo College (Florida) faculty in 1989. He holds a Bachelor of Science in Health Education from the University of Southern Mississippi, a Master of Arts in Health Education, and a Doctorate in Higher Education Administration, specializing in evaluation research, from the University of Florida. He has published over 20 articles in the areas of public health, health program administration, and health professions education. His research interests are community health analysis and the evaluation of primary prevention programs. Prior to joining Saint Leo College, Dr. Hale worked for 10 years in public health as a service provider, institutional researcher, and program administrator. Dr. Hale has consulted with state and national organizations.

Frank Arnold, Associate Professor of Management and Public Administration, joined the faculty of Saint Leo College in September, 1988. He holds a Bachelor of Science in Business Administration from the University of Connecticut, a Master of Public Administration from Auburn University, and a Doctorate in Public Administration from Nova University. Since 1981, he has taught at five different institutions as either a full-time or adjunct professor. Prior to joining Saint Leo College, Dr. Arnold worked in industry as a senior systems analyst. Prior to that, he retired as a Colonel from the United States Air Force after a 25 year career.

Marvin T. Travis, Professor of Management, became Dean of the Division of Business Administration at Saint Leo College in 1984 after joining the faculty in 1982. Dr. Travis holds a Bachelor of Arts in Economics from Emory University, a Master of Business Administration from Arizona State University, and a Doctorate in Public Administration from Nova University. Before joining Saint Leo College, Dr. Travis served 23 years in the United States Air Force and five years as a faculty member with the University of Tampa. Dr. Travis is a consultant to business, government, and health care organizations.

SECTION *I*

Operations Health Program Planning and Evaluation

1

The Planning Challenge

Chapter Objective:

1. Describe the strategic management process.

The most important responsibility of the manager is to plan. In the management literature, the lists of managerial functions consistently begin with planning and always include that function regardless of the number of other managerial functions that may be listed and described.

If planning is so important, should it be assumed that the top manager in any enterprise gives this primary attention? The answer is no. The paradox of the typical promotion ladder is that the top executive position goes to someone who has been successful as a person of action in the daily give-and-take of crisis management. In fact, there has usually been little training in the typical business for the individual who will assume the top position.

Over the past twenty years, management theorists have given increasing attention to the subject of planning. Much of the decline in the competitiveness of American industry has been attributed to the managerial obsession with the next income statement and balance sheet. Seldom do senior managers consider the long-term effectiveness of an organization beyond their tenure. Senior management's rewards are usually determined by the earnings per share of stock in a given year. In the non-profit sector, rewards are allocated for staying within budget. The reward system should consider how effective the firm will be in the next five to ten years.

An example of a short-term management focus is the repeating cycle of nursing shortages. The shortage of nurses is not just the result of poor pay, but the lack of true professional recognition, lack of decision-making authority, poor working conditions, and rotation policies that increase stress and lead to burn-out. Senior managers frequently blame tight budgets as the cause, yet there has been practically no planning by these same managers to solve the problem. So, the cycle continues.

STRATEGIC MANAGEMENT: AN INTRODUCTION _____

If managers have been poor planners in the past, the growing attention given to the concept of Strategic Management provides a means to improve performance. Rue and Holland (1989, p. 3) describe strategic management as "the process by which top management determines the long-run direction and performance of the organization by ensuring that careful formulation, proper implementation, and continuous evaluation of the strategy takes place." Strategic management implies long-term management. In turn, the strategy (i.e., a comprehensive, integrated organization-wide plan also referred to as a strategic plan) is put into place as the result of the strategic management process. In effect, a strategy defines the way an entire organization will achieve its stated goals and objectives. The attainment of these goals and objectives is essential for organizational success, i.e., accomplishing its mission.

Levels of Strategic Management

Strategic management is a process that should involve the entire organization. Participation by all levels in the organization will result in improved acceptance of the resulting organizational strategy and, hence, improve the chances of organizational success. Also, managers throughout the organization are a valuable resource in determining the proper direction for strategic improvement. Thus, the strategic management process involves several levels where action is required:

a. *Corporate level:* At this level (e.g., a multi-hospital system), the top executive officers decide and communicate the long-term mission of the entire organization. They coordinate and approve lower level plans and exercise control over key elements of the strategic plan that require their personal attention. Key elements are those that must be successful if the organization is to survive.
b. *Strategic business unit (SBU) level:* The general manager, who usually has total authority for the operation of a subsidiary of the corporation (e.g., a hospital operated by the hospital system) and who develops subordinate plans which support planning at the corporate level.
c. *Functional level:* The director of a specialized service, (e.g., the hospital's medical records department) and who develops plans which support those of the SBU.
d. *Operational level:* Here, a first-line supervisor (e.g., the supervisor of the utilization review section of the medical records department) develops plans that support the broader plans of those levels above the operating unit.

A second example is presented in Figure 1.1 for fictitious Cherry Hill Healthcare Systems. Strategic management levels are labeled.

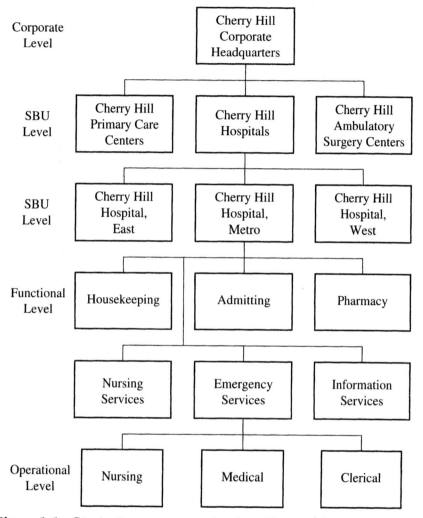

Figure 1.1 Strategic management levels at Cherry Hill Healthcare Systems, Inc.

Cherry Hill is a private, for-profit corporate system. Cherry Hill operates seven primary care centers, three hospitals, and four same-day-surgery centers in a large urban center. For the past three years, Cherry Hill has been enjoying increasing market share, service volume, and earnings per share. Cherry Hill is largely dependent upon Medicare; but its free-standing primary care and ambulatory surgery centers have been attracting a growing number of private and third party payors. These are considered SBUs.

Within the Cherry Hill Hospital SBU, there are three hospitals, each of which is independently responsible for its own profit or loss. Each hospital is also a SBU. For example, Cherry Hill Metro Hospital has several departments which are at the functional level. Six are presented in Figure 1.1. Each department's operations planning must support that of the hospital.

Within each department are sections, teams, or shifts. In the Emergency Services Department are three sections: medical, nursing, and clerical. Planning activities conducted within each section must support those of the department.

As one moves down the system hierarchy, planning activities become increasingly operational in nature to the point of affecting a single section, or shift, within a department. As one moves up the system hierarchy, planning activities become increasingly broad and applicable to the system (or organization) as a whole.

In many ways, planning at operations levels is more difficult, as the supervisor must integrate his or her planning with the levels above. However, when the plans of each of these levels are integrated into a comprehensive organizational strategy (or strategic plan), the organization is better positioned to achieve its stated goals and objectives, and hence, its mission.

It is at the operations level that a manager's career in the important process of planning usually begins. A knowledge of the way in which operations planning fits into the entire strategic management system demonstrates the importance of the subject if an organization is to be successful.

✳ The Typical Strategic Management Process

Strategic management is a dynamic, constantly evolving process, whereby all organizational elements are being assessed at the same time. Planning activity is guided by evaluation results garnered from the implementation of plans. Although we may devise a linear relationship to describe the specific parts of the process, it is probably more accurate to compare the process to a spinning ball moving through space. This is because the process is continually repeating itself with different activities occurring at the same time. There is general consensus among those who have written and consulted in the area of strategic management on the process to be followed. The following outline is typical:

a. Define the business and establish the strategic mission for ultimate accomplishment. *Results in mission Statement* *Corp*
b. Evaluate present strategy as well as current and past performance. *level*
c. Evaluate the environment to determine opportunities and threats. Study social, economic, technological, competitor, supplier, and governmental sectors.
d. Analyze the internal strengths and weaknesses of the organization. Study finance, operations, marketing, personnel, and technological capacities.
e. Establish long-range goals and shorter-range objectives that will lead to the accomplishment of the goals at all levels within the organization, thus, achieving the organization's mission.

f. Evaluate alternative means of achieving the goals and objectives and choose the best alternative course of action.

g. Develop the strategic plan for implementation throughout the organization including functional and operating levels of the organization.

h. Establish a formal evaluation process in all key areas to monitor performance. Make changes in the plans as necessary to ensure goals and objectives are met.

While a detailed discussion of the strategic management process is beyond the scope of this book, a brief discussion of each phase of the process is presented below in order to familiarize you with the process:

Eval policies Constantly Once Instituted

a. *Define the business and establish the strategic mission for ultimate accomplishment.* Within this phase, a large system or a single organization will determine what is its reason for existence (i.e., its mission statement). Thus, the mission statement is central to all systems or organizational activity. In our present example, Cherry Hill determined that its mission was to provide comprehensive healthcare services in a cost efficient manner so as to maintain the system's financial viability, hence, Cherry Hill organized three SBUs: primary care centers, hospitals, and same-day-surgery centers.

b.. *Evaluate present strategy as well as current and past performance.* It appears that Cherry Hill has met with some success. Over the past three years, the corporation has experienced significant increases in market share, service volume, and profitability. Thus, Cherry Hill's strategy of three SBUs, each targeting a specific segment of the area's healthcare market, has been successful. Further, Cherry Hill routinely monitors its external environment for opportunities and threats and its internal environment for strengths and weaknesses.

c.. *Evaluate the environment to determine opportunities and threats. Study social, economic, technological, competitor, supplier, and governmental sectors.* Cherry Hill's management has conducted external environmental reviews involving each of the sectors mentioned above. For example, the governmental relations specialist predicted the repeal of Medicare's catastrophic health care insurance program. The repeal of catastrophic health care insurance would reduce the system's hospital-derived income as Medicare reimbursement would be reduced. The ambulatory care marketing specialist found that there was potential for increasing Cherry Hill's market share within the free-standing primary care product line.

d. *Analyze the internal strengths and weaknesses of the organization. Study finance, operations, marketing, personnel, and technological capacities.* Cherry Hill conducted a thorough internal environmental scan of its current finance, marketing, personnel, and technological resources as well as its administrative operations. The health planners found that the expected drop in hospital revenue would cause the system to have excess capacity and reduced average length of stay at two of the three hospitals. This, in turn, would lead to a surplus in administrative, medical, nursing, allied health, and clerical personnel. Further, an internal facilities analysis found that administrative operations, which had been located outside of each hospital, could be consolidated into each hospital, thus eliminating rental expenses.

e. *Establish long-range goals and shorter-range objectives that will lead to the accomplishment of the goals at all levels within the organization, thus, achieving the organization's mission.* Once the external and internal environmental analysis had been completed, line managers, with the assistance of the planning staff, began the process of developing objectives which supported the corporate goal of financial viability, as required by the mission statement.

f. *Evaluate alternative means of achieving the goals and objectives and choose the best alternative course of action.* Corporate health planners evaluated several alternatives that would allow the corporation to achieve the goal of financial success as required by its mission statement. From the alternative strategies, one was selected which focused on: (a) expanding a profitable product line and (b) taking steps to eliminate expensive excess service capacity.

g. *Develop the strategic plan for implementation throughout the organization including functional and operating levels of the organization.* Within this phase, managers throughout the organization developed detailed plans to open two free-standing primary care clinics. Because each of the previous phases of the strategic management process was carefully conducted, Cherry Hill managers were able to shift human and material resources to an expanded product line (i.e., free-standing primary care centers) without personnel reductions and to reduce financial outlays for additional space. Of course, some clinical equipment and material would have to be purchased to equip and stock the two free-standing centers. All of this was done to meet the financial goal as required by the mission statement.

h. *Establish a formal evaluation process in all key areas to monitor performance. Make changes in the plans, as necessary, to ensure goals and objectives are met.* A variety of monitoring devices were used. They included regular staff meetings, progress reports, time lines, PERT charts, on-site visitation, financial ratio analysis, and the firm's computerized management information system. Any deviation from the prescribed plan was noted, investigated, corrected, and, where necessary, the plan was adjusted.

Managing the Process

There must be a strong commitment by top management to a strategic management process if it is to be successful. Most subordinate managers pay attention to what the boss says is important. Without the active participation and direction from the top, the planning effort will only receive token attention. Top management must devise a workable system of strategic planning and communicate that process and attendant time lines to ensure success. However, the approach must not only be top-down, but also bottom-up. Top managers should ask for and encourage ideas and recommendations that will become dynamic parts of the final organizational strategy from the lowest levels of the organization. The establishment of individual objectives for personal achievement, sometimes using a Management by Objectives (MBO) approach, will fit neatly into the process of developing a corporate-wide strategic plan.

Many large organizations have professional planners on staff to assist in the direction of the planning effort. The staff planner may well direct the overall administration of a planning cycle. The planner will probably set suspense (due) dates for all managers to meet. However, such planners should always be in an advisory (i.e., staff) role; they should not direct or replace the planning activity of line managers. The key player remains the line manager at all levels. *Must have last word in what will occur.*

The literature of strategic management is replete with strong evidence that those organizations that have a formal system of strategic planning are more successful than those that do not formally plan. Since a manager's first exposure to planning is usually at the operations level, the focus of the following chapters is on those elements of planning that will be most useful to the operations oriented manager.

SUMMARY

Strategic management is a process by which organizations order their management and planning efforts. Organizations that fail to systematically plan are more likely to fail in achieving their goals and objectives.

There are four levels of strategic management: corporate, strategic business unit, functional, and operational. Planning occurs at each level. As one moves from the corporate to the operations level, planning becomes increasingly centered about day-to-day business activities.

A strategic management system is a process of eight interdependent phases. Each phase supports the others and occurs within each strategic level of the organization. When operating correctly, a comprehensive strategic management system will improve an organization's performance.

REVIEW QUESTIONS

1. What is the most important responsibility of a manager?
   a. Organize
   b. Plan
   c. Lead
   d. Control

2. Senior managerial reward systems should consider which one of the following?
   a. Annual net income
   b. Quarterly profits
   c. The income statement
   d. Long-term effectiveness

3. The definition, "the process by which top management determines the long-run direction and performance of the organization . . ." refers to which one of the following?
   a. Strategic mission
   b. Strategic management
   c. Strategic planning
   d. Operations planning

4. Organizational success is to achieve:
   a. Goals
   b. Objectives
   c. Mission
   d. "b" and "c"

5. When the top executive officers of an organization develop the direction which the organization will follow, which level of the strategic management team is most likely involved?
   a. Corporate
   b. SBU
   c. Functional
   d. Operational

6. Within a multi-hospital system which operates in three states, an independent regional CEO (who is responsible for total operations in a single state) would likely be at which one of the following strategic planning levels?
   a. Corporate
   b. SBU
   c. Functional
   d. Operational

7. Within a multi-hospital system which operates in three states, first line supervisors would likely be at which one of the following strategic planning levels?
   a. Corporate
   b. SBU
   c. Functional
   d. Operational

8. If a strategic management process is to work within an organization, certain principles must be closely followed. All of the following are considered to be included within those principles EXCEPT:
   a. A strong commitment by top management must be exhibited.
   b. It is best if most planning efforts flow bottom-up and top-down.
   c. Objectives should be established for individuals to achieve.
   d. With respect to planning, line managers should have a staff role.

9. Typically, most top managers are appointed because of their strategic management and planning abilities.
   a. True
   b. False

10. In health services organizations, most managers are first exposed to planning at which strategic management level?
    a. Corporate
    b. SUB
    c. Functional
    d. Operational

DISCUSSION QUESTIONS

1. Select an organization with which you are familiar. Identify the various strategic management levels within it and describe how each level plans for the future.

2. Select an organization and analyze its strategic management processes using the model outlined in this chapter. How are the processes similar and dissimilar?

3. Describe the ideal relationship between a staff planner and a manager. In a small organization, how might these roles be combined?

Teamwork, Displomacy

2

An Operations Health Program Planning Model

Chapter Objectives:

1. Describe the operations health program.
2. Describe the operations health program planning model.

Robbins (1991, p. 194) defined operational plans as "plans that specify how overall objectives [i.e., goals] are to be achieved." Operations planning develops the means to implement an organization's strategic planning goals.

Operations health planning is conducted by operations oriented managers who are positioned close to those points within a health care and health related organization where goods and services are produced and/or delivered. Operations planning usually does not extend beyond one to three years and is narrowly focused as compared to strategic planning whose planning horizon may extend to as much as five to seven years or even further into the future.

THE PLANNING PROCESS

From our vantage point, planning is a sequence of eight steps, or phases, which are:

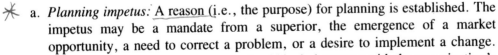

a. *Planning impetus:* A reason (i.e., the purpose) for planning is established. The impetus may be a mandate from a superior, the emergence of a market opportunity, a need to correct a problem, or a desire to implement a change. Whatever the reason or purpose, it should be in harmony with the organization's mission statement.

b. *Acquiring knowledge:* Those involved in the planning effort may need to acquire knowledge about the reason for planning, the subject involved, or the planning process. It is always advisable to learn as much as possible. Not only will the manager be better prepared, but a higher quality plan will emerge. (Chapters 5, 6, 7, and 8 are intended to help you acquire and interpret information useful in health planning.)

c. *Developing and selecting broad options:* Within this phase, broad options, designed to achieve the stated purpose of the plan, are researched and evaluated (according to whatever criteria have been established). The result of this process is usually a single goal or a few goals, depending on the scope of the plan.

d. *Developing the general means to accomplish selected options:* Once the broad options have been selected, the general means (e.g., objectives) for accomplishing each option are developed. During this phase, it may be necessary to revise goals and/or acquire additional information in order to specify attainable objectives. Once developed, objectives are subsumed under the corresponding goal.

e. *Developing detailed specifications for accomplishing each selected option:* Once the general framework is in place, detailed specifications (called activities and/or service targets) are developed. These are then subsumed under the corresponding objective. When combined, a draft plan emerges. (A full documentation model is presented in Chapter 4.)

f. *Plan is submitted for approval:* In this phase, the draft plan is reviewed and refined by the planner, a planning committee, or peers. The plan is revised as needed. Next, the planner may formally present the plan or simply deliver it to the approving authority. Once approval has been obtained, the plan is ready for implementation. (The discussion in Chapter 9 may be helpful in developing a strategy for obtaining plan approval.)

g. *Plan implementation:* At this point, the plan is implemented. It may be necessary to adjust the implementation schedule, or even the plan, given field experience. You should not be afraid to do this if warranted. Be sure to consult with the relevant superior(s) and/or subordinate(s). (The discussion in Chapter 9 may assist during this phase.)

h. *Plan monitoring and necessary adjustment:* This phase actually begins during implementation and extends throughout the life span of the plan. The program or project is then monitored to ensure compliance with plan provisions and/or identify areas where adjustments are needed. The successful execution of this phase relies heavily on the plan's evaluation element (Chapter 3) and its management information system (Chapters 10 and 11).

The operational planning process is summarized in Figure 2.1. The two-way arrows signify that the border between each step is blurred, as it is often necessary to go back and forth between steps before moving on to the next.

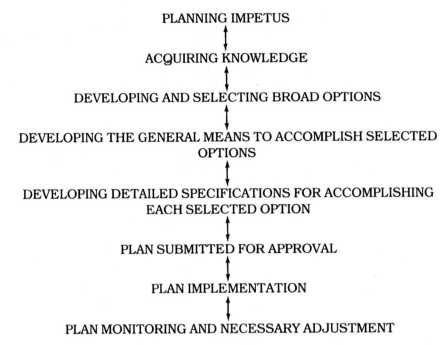

Figure 2.1   An operations planning model

"Building Blocks" of Planning

Organizations exist for specific reasons. These reasons are contained in the organization's mission statement. In order to achieve its mission, an organization should develop goals which are supported by very specific objectives. Objectives are, in turn, supported by activities and service targets. Taken together, the mission statement, goals, objectives, activities, and service targets are the building blocks of health planning.

The following terms, (mission, goal, objective, and service target) are defined as follows:

Know for Quiz

Mission:	"the purpose of an organization" (Robbins, 1991, p. 220).
Goal:	"a long-range specified state of accomplishment toward which programs are directed" (Reinke, 1988, p. 67).
Objective:	"stated in terms of achieving a measured amount of progress toward a goal, specifies:
what:	the nature of the situation or condition to be attained.
how much:	the quantity or amount of the situation or condition to be attained.
when:	the time at or by which the desired situation or condition is intended to exist.

_ *who:* the particular group of people or portion of the environment in which attainment is desired, and,

where: the geographic area to be included in the program" (Reinke, 1988, p. 67).

Service
Target: specifies level of service volume directed towards a defined target population.

Activity: action steps which must be executed in order to achieve a specified objective.

These "building blocks," when operationalized, are sequenced within the operations health program planning process presented in Figure 2.2. *← Employers*

While not a "building block," *performance standards* are essential in operations health planning as they determine what is the acceptable level of productivity each worker is to render. Objectives, service targets, and activities, therefore, are dependent on reasonable, specified employee performance standards, which are often written into employee job or position descriptions.

✳ Comments Concerning Objectives

While there are many approaches to planning, the present model employs as objective attainment approach. Within this approach, measurable objectives are established, towards which effort is expended. Objectives provide focus, direction, and degree of attainment indication. Such an approach is easy to understand, utilize, implement, monitor, and evaluate. There are different types of objectives depending on what is to be accomplished. These objectives are: (a) outcome objectives, (b) process objectives, and (c) management objectives.

Health programs should have *outcome objectives*, which are usually for the duration of the program (for most grant funded programs three to five years is the maximum funding period). The attainment of outcome objectives yields the best evidence that the program has accomplished its goal(s) insofar as possible given available funding, staffing, and prevailing conditions. If a program's goal is written as an objective and the program is of limited duration, such a goal could substitute for an outcome objective. Please note that some health programs use outcome objectives to describe a program's impact on a population's health status, disease prevalence, or disease incidence. For an example, see the goal for the Hardee Cog Company case in this chapter.

In addition to management objectives, health programs may have *process objectives* (in small programs or projects, service targets and/or activities may substitute) which are up to one year in length (but usually less) and are monitored monthly or quarterly. The attainment of process objectives ensures that the program is on the course necessary to meet the program's goal(s). Process objectives are concerned with such things as incremental service delivery, which when fully delivered, will lead to outcome objective attainment.

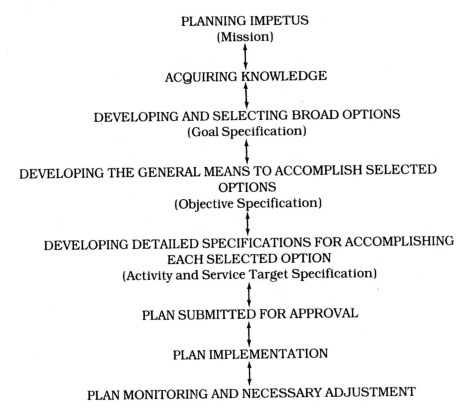

PLANNING IMPETUS
(Mission)

↑

ACQUIRING KNOWLEDGE

↑

DEVELOPING AND SELECTING BROAD OPTIONS
(Goal Specification)

↑

DEVELOPING THE GENERAL MEANS TO ACCOMPLISH SELECTED
OPTIONS
(Objective Specification)

↑

DEVELOPING DETAILED SPECIFICATIONS FOR ACCOMPLISHING
EACH SELECTED OPTION
(Activity and Service Target Specification)

↑

PLAN SUBMITTED FOR APPROVAL

↑

PLAN IMPLEMENTATION

↑

PLAN MONITORING AND NECESSARY ADJUSTMENT

Figure 2.2   Integrated operations planning model

Each health program and/or project should have a *management objective,* whose attainment ensures smooth program operation. These management objectives should normally be a year in duration, with monthly or quarterly monitoring. Management objectives are concerned with such things as reports to the funding agency, employee activities (e.g., selection, training and evaluation), program support activities (e.g., office equipment and supplies), and promotional activities (e.g., newsletters, speaker's bureau, etc.). To achieve efficient and effective monitoring, each program or project should be part of a management information system (MIS). If you are unfamiliar with management information systems, you may find Chapters 10 and 11 instructive.

INTEGRATED OPERATIONS HEALTH
PLANNING MODEL

We will now examine an integrated operational health planning model (Figure 2.2). Subsumed under selected stages of the planning process are the "building blocks" mentioned earlier. It is within these stages, that the "building blocks" are formed and laid. For example, the final output of developing and selecting broad options is the program's goal. In the same manner, the final output of developing the general means to accomplish the selected option(s) are the program's objectives.

PLANNING: A POLITICAL AND
TECHNICAL PROCESS

Table 2.1 has been developed to communicate which steps of the operations planning process are technical and/or political. Presented in the third column is the dominant activity and/or physical outcome of each stage of the operations health planning model. As you can see, health planning (or any other type of planning) has a fairly systematic and technical base. However, the planner or planning committee that fails to take into account institutional politics is doomed to difficulty or failure. The information presented in Chapter 9 may be helpful when dealing with institutional politics.

The reason that the political stages of the planning process have been pointed out is that there is a need to remember to consult appropriate formal and informal leaders, affected constituencies, involved decision makers, and other relevant publics. Such

Table 2.1 Operational planning model, task type, & dominant activity

Planning Model	Task	Dominant Activity
1. Planning Impetus	Political & Technical	This can be a response to a mandate or other stimulus.
2. Acquiring Knowledge	Technical	Conduct research.
3. Developing and Selecting Broad Options	Political & Technical	Statement of program goal(s) is final outcome.
4. Developing the General Means to Accomplish Selected Options	Political & Technical	Statement of program objectives is outcome.
5. Developing Detailed Specifications for Accomplishing Each Selected Option	Technical	Statement of activities, service targets, & support requirements is outcome.
6. Plan Submitted for Approval	Political & Technical	Negotiation and compromise may be required.
7. Plan Implementation	Political & Technical	Each plan should have an implementation period.
8. Plan Monitoring and Necessary Adjustment	Technical	Done by monitoring MIS reports and doing program evaluation.

✗ A-f

consultation has several advantages, which include: (a) later opposition tends to be lessened; (b) excellent ideas are often offered, which enhance the quality and relevance of the proposed program or project; (c) potential adversaries very often become supporters; (d) democratic ideals are reinforced; (e) target populations tend to become empowered to provide for themselves; and (f) the prospects for approval and implementation are improved.

Case: Hardee Cog Company, Inc.

Effective November 1, 1992, you along with 2 other operations (i.e., line) managers and 2 non-managerial employees have been appointed to a planning group by the president of Hardee Cog Company. The president has charged your group with developing an employee wellness plan for the company. However, since Hardee Cog has no experience with employee wellness plans, your team has been instructed to keep the initial program plan modest but fully staffed should the company decide to undertake other activities. The team has been given two months (November and December, 1992) to plan the program plan.

Your team is to (a) review the company's mission statement, (b) review an employee health behavior survey results printout (Appendix 2.A), (c) formulate a project goal to be achieved, (d) specify an appropriate number of objectives, and (e) outline service targets and activities sufficient to achieve the stated objectives. This case will be further developed.

Hardee Cog Corporate Mission Statement:

The Corporate Mission of Hardee Cog is to produce high quality cogs and make a positive contribution to the welfare of our customers, employees and home community as well as provide exceptional financial returns to stockholders.

Hardee Cog Employee Wellness Planning Group's Goal:

The Employee Wellness Planning Group will design a demonstration employee wellness program based on the consultant's report of employee health behaviors which was commissioned by the Hardee Cog Executive Committee.

The Human Resources Department has reported that three employees were killed and 18 corporate family members have been injured due to automobile accidents where seatbelts were not used during the past 16 months. The company is self-insured and the health care costs have nearly depleted the company's insurance fund. The Human Resources Department conducted a survey of health related behaviors that included seatbelt use.

After reviewing the survey results (Apppendix 2.A), the planning team has decided to target employee lack of seatbelt use. The following data are contained within the printout:

Seatbelt Use	(#) Frequency	(%) Respondents
Never	2	0.25
Seldom	411	52.20
Sometimes	117	14.83
Nearly Always	162	20.53
Always	97	12.28

Getting people to change seatbelt use behaviors generally requires little inconvenience on the part of the target population (hence a greater likelihood of program success) and is a fairly easy program to implement. Your planning team has developed the following goal, objectives, service targets, and activities:

Program Goal:

To increase the percentage of employees who always wear seatbelts from 12% to 75%, with seatbelt preventable injuries halved by 15 October 1993. (Could Substitute as an Outcome Objective)

Program Objectives: *Breakouts of Goal*

1. To mandate the use of seatbelts 100% of the time by occupants riding or driving in company owned or rented vehicles effective 1 February 1993. (Process Objective)
2. To have 90% of employees attend a seatbelt education session and score at least 75% of correct answers on a quiz by 1 September 1993. (Process Objective)
3. To have 90% of employees report positive attitudes towards seatbelt use on a written survey instrument by 30 September 1993. (Process Objective)
4. To effectively and efficiently manage the company's project between 1 November 1992 and 31 October 1993. (Management Objective)

Program Service Targets and Activities: *Breakouts Objectives*

Objective 1   To mandate the use of seatbelts 100% of the time by occupants riding or driving in company owned or rented vehicles effective 1 February 1993.

Subparts of objectives

1a. Propose that the president mandate a company-wide seatbelt use policy with a non-compliance sanction by 10 January 1993.
1b. Testify before the Corporate Executive Committee as to the advantages of such a policy at the 15 January 1993 meeting.
1c. Once the policy has been adopted, disseminate the policy to employees through payroll distribution by 25 January 1993.

Objective 2   To have 90% of employees attend a seatbelt education session and score at least 75% of correct answers on a quiz by 1 September 1993.

2a. Develop an educational curriculum to educate employees about the advantages of seatbelt use by 1 March 1993.
2b. Schedule, advertise, and initiate education sessions (advise supervisors to count as time worked session attendance) between 1 April and 1 September 1993.
2c. Conduct 20 educational sessions (20 sessions with an average of 40 participants) by 1 September 1993.
2d. Conduct ten free educational sessions for employee families and interested community members by 1 September 1993.

Objective 3   To have 90% of employees report positive attitudes towards seatbelt use on a written survey instrument by 30 September 1993.

3a. Post five different seatbelt use posters, monthly, in each of ten departments starting in November 1992 for 12 months.
3b. Distribute a seatbelt reminder with each employee pay check between 1 January and 31 October 1993.
3c. Publish the names of employees who are found wearing seatbelts in company vehicles, thus making them eligible for periodic drawings for free gifts to be conducted quarterly between 1 January and 31 October 1993.
3d. Operate a free seatbelt information table using educational literature between 1 January and 31 October 1993.
3e. Distribute free bumper stickers to employees and make employees who display the sticker eligible for cash prizes to be awarded quarterly between 1 January and 31 October 1993.
3f. Employ a consultant to conduct an employee survey to ascertain and report employee attitudes and behaviors concerning seatbelt use by 30 September 1993.

Objective 4   To efficiently and effectively manage the company's project between 1 November 1992 and 31 October 1993.

4a. Report to the Corporate Executive Committee quarterly between 1 November 1992 and 31 October 1993.

4b. Employ staff by 31 December 1992.

4c. Report implementation evaluation results by 1 March 1993.

4d. Report to the Corporate Executive Committee the final impact evaluation results by 31 October 1993.

4e. Design, conduct, and report a comprehensive needs analysis addressing employee wellness and disease prevention needs by 31 October 1993.

Diagraming Objectives

Often it is helpful to "diagram" objectives when writing them. This is done by taking each definition component and then "filling-in-the-blank." This has been done for each objective presented above. Once you have filled in all the "blanks," you will nearly have your objectives written.

Objective 1   To mandate the use of seatbelts 100% of the time by occupants riding or driving in company owned or rented vehicles effective 1 February 1993.

> *What:* mandated use of seatbelts
> *How much:* 100% of the time
> *When:* by 1 February 1993
> *Who:* occupants
> *Where:* riding or driving in company owned or rented vehicles

Objective 2   To have 90% of employees attend a seatbelt education session and score at least 75% of correct answers on a quiz by 1 September 1993.

> *What:* attend seatbelt education sessions and score correct answers on a quiz
> *How Much:* 90% employee attendance and 75% correct answers
> *When:* by 1 September 1993
> *Who:* employees
> *Where:* on company property (Implied)

Objective 3   To have 90% of employees report positive attitudes towards seatbelt use on a written survey instrument by 30 September 1993.

> *What:* report positive attitudes
> *How Much:* 90%
> *When:* by 30 September 1993

Who: employees
Where: on a written survey instrument

Objective 4   To efficiently and effectively manage the company's project between 1 November 1992 and 31 October 1993.

What: efficiently and effectively manage
How Much: 100% (Implied)
When: between 1 November 1992 and 30 October 1993
Who: program manager (Implied)
Where: company

The phrase "to efficiently and effectively manage" is intended to convey the message that it is the responsibility of management to ethically administer the plan's activities. Obviously such an assessment is based on an ex post facto analysis of a manager's decisions and actions. There are techniques that will assist a manager such as monthly or quarterly reports which describe "current" activity, service target, and objective attainment. Monthly or quarterly financial reports should also be utilized. In an era of scarce resources and an increased accountability, the authors strongly advocate the inclusion of a management objective for each plan. Such an objective should clearly detail what steps will be taken to efficiently and effectively manage resources.

Service Targets and Activities

Under each objective are listed service targets and activities, each with a unique identifier code. For the reader's convenience, a classification taxonomy is presented:

Activities	Service Targets
1a, 1b, 1c, 2a, 2b, 3b, 3c, 3d, 3e, 3f, 4a, 4b, 4c, 4d, & 4e	2c, 2d, & 3a

Usually, a service target spells out explicitly a specific service, the anticipated service level, to whom the service is being provided, and a date by which service delivery will be completed. Activities typically spell out specific actions that must be taken in order to accomplish an objective and a completion date only.

Sometimes it is hard to classify something as either an activity or service target. When this happens, ask yourself if there is any explicitly stated quantity of things being provided, service level stated, and an identifiable target group. If the answer to each is yes, then you have a service target. If the answer to each is no, then you have an activity. Study the examples on the previous pages.

The Gantt Chart

When objectives, activities, and service targets have associated time lines, it is a good idea to use a Gantt Chart. A Gantt Chart is a management device that helps a planner and/or program manager to efficiently and effectively manage program operations. A sample Gantt Chart has been developed for the above case. See Figure 2.3. See also the two cases in Section IV.

The objective, service target, and/or activity unique identifier codes are placed on the vertical axis. The months and years included within the planning horizon are placed on the horizontal axis. Within the chart, mark the corresponding completion dates or coverage period dates for each objective, service target, or activity listed.

For example, when implemented, Objective 1 will cover the length of the program which extends between 10 January 1993 and 31 October 1993. Objective 1 attainment is

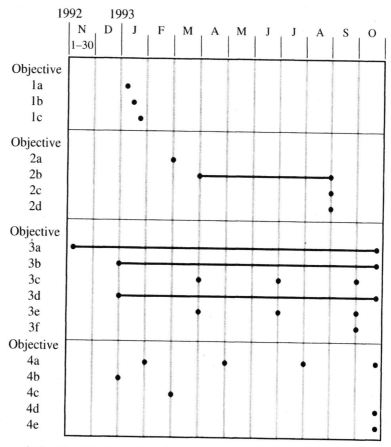

Figure 2.3 Gantt chart for the hardee cog employee seatbelt education program

predicated on activities 1a, 1b, and 1c, which have their own sequential time lines. Objectives 2, 3, and 4 are formatted in the same manner. Remember that while all objectives and service targets will have associated time lines, sometimes activities may not. However, we encourage all those engaging in planning to make sure that all activities have associated time lines, which makes managing program operations easier.

The advantages of using a Gantt Chart include:

a. The planner can ensure that sequential events are organized and timed to achieve successful completion;
b. The planner can determine whether the program's objectives are achievable within the program's planning horizon, (i.e., available time frame); and
c. The planner can evaluate whether objectives, activities, and/or service targets need to be added, deleted, or modified to achieve the program's goal.

SUMMARY

It is at the operations level where most managers are first exposed to planning. The planning process can be thought of as a series of steps which should be followed in sequence. Each operations level health plan should contain at least one goal which is supportive of the organization's mission statement. A goal should be supported by a sufficient number of objectives, service targets, and activities. Objectives should specify what, how much, when, who, and where. Planning is a political and technical process. Managers who assume the role of planner should involve those affected by a plan in the planning process. Organizations which engage in formal planning, regardless of level, typically outperform those which do not. Planning is a very important managerial function.

Appendix 2.A

Hardee Cog Employee Health Behavior Survey Results

SPONSOR CODE: 3241   HARDEE COG COMPANY
DATE: 3 September 1992

Behavior	Frequency	(%) Respondents
SEAT BELT USE		
a. Never	2	0.25
b. Seldom	411	52.20
c. Sometimes	117	14.83
d. Nearly Always	162	20.53

Behavior	Frequency	(%) Respondents
e. Always	97	12.28
BLOOD PRESSURE		
a. Told by a physician more than once BP high		
1. Yes	413	52.34
2. No	376	47.66
b. BP presently normal		
1. Yes	700	88.72
2. No	89	11.28
EXERCISE		
a. Participate in aerobic exercise		
1. Yes	212	26.87
2. No	577	73.13
b. Participate in other exercise		
1. Yes	489	61.98
2. No	300	38.02
c. Exercise type		
1. Running	98	12.42
2. Cycling	127	16.10
3. Walking	172	21.80
4. Gardening	50	6.34
5. Weight lifting	6	0.76
6. Other	36	4.56
7. None	300	38.02
d. Frequency of exercise		
1. No times	300	38.02
2. <once/wk.	27	3.43
3. 1/wk	215	27.25
4. 2/wk	157	19.90
5. 3/wk	57	7.22
6. 4/wk	24	3.04
7. 5 or more/wk	9	1.14
e. Duration of exercise		
1. No times	300	38.02
2. <15 min.	199	25.22
3. 15–30 min.	41	5.20
4. 30–45 min.	78	9.89
5. 45–60 min.	67	8.49
6. 60–90 min.	60	7.60
7. >90 min.	44	5.58

Behavior	Frequency	(%) Respondents
DIET AND NUTRITION		
a. Add salt to food at table		
1. Most of the time	159	20.15
2. Sometimes	135	17.11
3. Rarely	495	62.74
b. Red meat consumption		
1. None/never	41	5.20
2. 1–2/wk	249	31.55
3. 3–4/wk	341	43.22
4. 5–6/wk	90	11.41
5. 7/wi	68	8.62
c. Degree of Obesity		
1. less than 100%	60	7.60
2. Ideal body weight	101	12.80
3. 101–109% IBW	347	43.98
4. 110–119% IBW	100	12.67
5. 120% + IBW	181	22.95
SMOKING		
a. Smoke now		
1. Yes	469	59.44
2. No	320	40.56
b. Daily cigarette consumption		
1. <10/day	71	15.14
2. 11–20/day	98	20.89
3. 21–30/day	200	42.64
4. 31–40/day	53	11.30
5. >41/day	47	10.03
c. Stopped smoking for wk or more		
1. Yes	140	29.85
2. No	329	70.15
ALCOHOL		
a. Drink 2 or more drinks daily		
1. Don't drink or drink <2/day	413	52.34
2. 1–2 days/wk	102	12.93
3. 3–4 days/wk	89	11.28
4. 5–6 days/wk	50	6.34
5. 7 days/wk	135	17.11
b. Number of times drank 5 or more times/ occasion in past month		
1. Don't drink or drink <5/occasion	690	87.45

Behavior	Frequency	(%) Respondents
2. 1–2 occasions	47	5.96
3. 3–4 occasions	21	2.66
4. 5 or more	31	3.93
c. Driven when had too much		
1. Don't drink or drive while drinking	764	96.83
2. 1–2 times	18	2.28
3. 3–4 times	2	0.25
4. 5 or more	5	0.63
CHRONIC DISEASE MORBIDITY		
a. Diabetes Mellitus	40	5.10
b. Heart attack	43	5.45
c. HBP	87	11.03
d. Stroke	21	2.66
e. Alcoholism	71	9.00
f. Cancer or Leukemia	5	0.63
g. Drug Abuse	17	2.15
FOR WOMEN ONLY		
a. Most recent Pap Smear		
1. Never	3	0.57
2. Within past year	164	31.06
3. Within past 2 yrs.	232	43.94
4. Within past 3 yrs.	71	13.45
5. 4 or more yrs. ago	58	10.98
b. Family hist. Breast Ca.		
1. Yes	191	36.17
2. No	337	63.83
c. Practice monthly BSE		
1. Yes	89	16.86
2. No	439	83.14
a. Age		
1. <17	12	1.52
2. 18–24	59	7.48
3. 25–34	93	11.78
4. 35–44	186	23.57
5. 45–54	184	23.32
6. 55–64	170	21.56
7. 65+	85	10.77
b. Race		
1. White	767	97.22
2. Black	17	2.15

Behavior	Frequency	(%) Respondents
3. Other	5	0.63
c. Sex		
1. Male	261	33.08
2. Female	528	66.92
d. Education		
1. Less than 8th	33	4.18
2. Some high school	89	11.28
3. High school grad.	235	29.78
4. Some tech. sch.	28	3.55
5. Tech. sch. grad.	28	3.55
6. Some college	170	21.55
7. College grad.	123	15.59
8. Post grad. work	78	9.89
9. Refused	5	0.63
e. Marital Status		
1. Married	507	64.26
2. Widowed	128	16.22
3. Divorced	60	7.60
4. Never married	68	8.62
5. Refused	26	3.30
f. Occupation		
1. Managerial	90	11.41
2. Technical	77	9.76
3. Clerical	89	11.28
4. Production	516	65.40
5. Other	17	2.15
g. Household members		
1. 1–3 members	501	63.49
2. 4–6 members	200	25.36
3. 7+	88	11.15
h. Household income		
1. <10,000	110	13.95
2. 10–14,999	117	14.83
3. 15–19,999	106	13.43
4. 20–24,999	159	20.15
5. 25–34,999	93	11.79
6. 35,000+	91	11.53
7. Unknown	113	14.32

REVIEW AND APPLICATION QUESTIONS _____

1. This type of planning provides a general framework for the organization's movement into the future:
   a. Policy planning
   b. Program planning
   c. Strategic planning
   d. Operations planning

2. This type of planning is directed towards day-to-day activities of the organization:
   a. Policy planning
   b. Program planning
   c. Strategic planing
   d. Operations planning

3. Which term describes an organization's reason(s) for existence?
   a. Goal
   b. Mission
   c. Policy
   d. Objective

4. Which term describes a long-range specified state of accomplishment toward which efforts are directed?
   a. Goal
   b. Mission
   c. Policy
   d. Objective

5. Which one of the following is stated in terms of achieving a measured amount of progress towards a goal?
   a. Service target
   b. Performance standard
   c. Objective
   d. Activity

6. Which one of the following establishes a measured amount of output to be achieved in relation to a specific objective?
   a. Service target
   b. Performance standard
   c. Objective
   d. Activity

7. Which one of the following establishes an acceptable level of productivity a worker is to produce?
   a. Service target
   b. Performance standard
   c. Objective
   d. Activity

8. Which one of the following is an action which must be executed in order to achieve a specified objective?
   a. Service target
   b. Performance standard
   c. Objective
   d. Activity

9. Operations planning typically includes:
   a. 1–3 years
   b. 3–5 years
   c. 1 year
   d. 5 years

10. Which phase of the planning model produces a statement of program goal(s)?
    a. Developing broad options
    b. General means to accomplish selected options
    c. Plan implementation
    d. Detailed means for accomplishing selected options

11. Which phase of the planning model produces a statement of program objectives?
    a. Developing broad options
    b. General means to accomplish selected options
    c. Plan implementation
    d. Detailed means for accomplishing selected options

12. Which phase of the planning model produces a statement of activities and service targets?
    a. Developing broad options
    b. General means to accomplish selected options
    c. Plan implementation
    d. Detailed means for accomplishing selected options

13. The phase of the planning model where negotiation and compromise may be required is:
    a. Planning impetus
    b. Plan approval submission
    c. Plan implementation
    d. Acquiring knowledge

14. On a Gantt Chart, the program's unique identifier codes are listed on (the):
    a. Horizontal axis   c. Either axis
    b. Vertical axis   d. Within the grid

15. An objective whose attainment ensures that a program is on course towards its goal, but usually lasts less than one year, is called:
    a. A management objective
    b. A process objective
    c. An outcome objective
    d. An efficient objective

16. An objective whose attainment yields the best evidence of goal accomplishment is called:
    a. A management objective
    b. A process objective
    c. An outcome objective
    d. An efficient objective

17. Advantages of a Gantt Chart include all of the following EXCEPT:
    a. Assists in ensuring sequential events are organized to achieve completion
    b. Assists in determining if objectives are achievable within a given planning horizon
    c. Assists in determining whether or not objective, service target, performance standard, and activity adjustment is needed
    d. "a" and "b" are the only advantages

Questions 18 to 23 are related You sit on the planning committee for XYZ Hospital, which is an urban health center. The hospital has decided to develop a satellite family planning laboratory at one of its walk-in clinics. The lab is scheduled to open May 1, 1992. Identify each of the following statements.

18. XYZ Hospital will provide the most advanced health care at the least possible cost in a caring environment.
    a. Service target   c. Objectives
    b. Goal   d. Mission statement

19. XYZ Hospital will acquire, maintain, and utilize the latest diagnostic laboratory equipment.
    a. Mission statement   c. Goal
    b. Objective   d. Service target

20. XYZ Hospital's Family Planning Laboratory will correctly process at least 600 laboratory tests weekly by 1 June 1992.
    a. Goal   c. Service target
    b. Mission statement   d. Objective

21. XYZ Hospital's Family Planning Laboratory will process at least 200 pregnancy tests weekly.
    a. Performance standard c. Service target
    b. Objective   d. Goal

22. Each of the four family planning laboratory employees will correctly process 50 pregnancy tests weekly.
    a. Objective   c. Performance standard
    b. Service target   d. Activity

23. XYZ Hospital's Family Planning Laboratory will open at 1:00 pm and close at 5:00 pm daily.
    a. Activity   c. Objective
    b. Performance standard d. Service target

Questions 24 to 30 are related You sit on the planning committee for XYZ Hospital's employee wellness program. The planning committee has developed a nutrition education program. The program starts on 1 July 1991 and ends on 30 June 1992; identify each of the following statements.

24. XYZ Hospital will provide a comprehensive nutrition education program on its campus which will be attended by 90% of its employees by 30 June 1992.
    a. Service target
    b. Objective
    c. Goal
    d. Mission statement

25. The XYZ Hospital nutrition education program will be effectively and efficiently administered between 1 July 1991 and 30 June 1992.
    a. Process objective
    b. Management objective
    c. Outcome objective
    d. Don't know

26. XYZ Hospital will provide the community, patients, and employees with the best health care at the least possible cost.
    a. Goal
    b. Mission statement
    c. Objective
    d. Activity

27. During the first shift, each nutrition education session will start at 10:00 am and end at 11:00 am.
    a. Performance standard
    b. Service target
    c. Activity
    d. Objective

28. XYZ Hospital will provide a safe, nurturing, and healthy work environment.
    a. Objective
    b. Mission statement
    c. Performance standard
    d. Goal

29. Each health educator will conduct an average of 18 nutrition education classes per month between 1 July 1991 and 30 June 1992.
    a. Objective
    b. Activity
    c. Performance standard
    d. Service target

30. The nutrition education program of XYZ Hospital will provide 12 (3 per shift) nutrition education classes to employees on healthy eating basics by 30 August 1991.
    a. Service target
    b. Performance standard
    c. Activity
    d. Objective

DISCUSSION QUESTIONS

1. Identify an organization about which you are knowledgeable. Analyze how that organization plans compared to the planning model discussed in this chapter.

2. Describe the difference between outcome, process, and management objectives.

3. Explain the difference between activities and service targets.

4. Explain why a Gantt Chart might be useful in a planning effort.

5. Select some data from Appendix 2.A and write a goal and supporting objectives, service targets, and activities.

3

A Program Evaluation Model

Chapter Objectives:

1. Describe the program evaluation model.
2. Describe an application of the program evaluation model.

For many, talking about evaluation is akin to announcing that the IRS is going to audit their tax return. Well, this doesn't have to be the case.

Evaluation, conducted as the program is implemented and operating, provides information which enables program managers to correct performance deficits and/or undesirable deviations from the expected course. When a program is evaluated, summatively, an opportunity to determine what worked within a program, what didn't, and why is afforded.

Examined within this chapter are: (a) the concept of evaluation, (b) an operations program evaluation model, and (c) selected issues in program evaluation. Since a detailed, technical discussion of health program evaluation is beyond the scope of this book, the interested reader is invited to examine Kosecoff and Fink (1982), Patton (1990), and Rubinson and Neutens (1987).

EVALUATION: AN INTRODUCTION

Purpose and Characteristics

Rubinson and Neutens (1987, p. 12) have defined evaluation research as "a method of evaluating a process to enable judgments to be more accurate and objective." Anderson, Ball, and Murphy (1981, pp. 136–137) have outlined a purpose and characteristics of program evaluation which include: (a) "to provide information for decisions about the program"; (b) "evaluation results should be useful for program-improvement decisions, not just for decisions about continuation or termination"; (c) "evaluation results should be provided in time to be useful for such decisions"; (d) "evaluation is a human judgmental process applied to results of program examination"; and (e) "evaluation should take into account the . . . objectives of the program." Also, when evaluating a program, one should document the observed, but unintended, effects of a health program.

Based on the above paragraph, we can see that evaluation is a type of research which is designed to produce timely information for use in making judgments concerning program improvement, management, and continuation. Thus, program evaluation is an important element in the planning of any health program. This is especially true in an environment which demands clear accountability for operational efficiency and effectiveness.

Relationship to Health Services Research

Evaluation can be viewed as an application of health services research methodology. The data collection, analysis, and reporting processes are the same. Evaluators, use demographic (Chapter 5), epidemiological (Chapter 6), health services (Chapter 7), and budgetary (Chapter 8) data. *frequency*

An important characteristic of evaluation research is that the results of an evaluation study are used to make judgments regarding a specific program, process, or event. Health service *may* involve such judgment, but evaluation research *must*.

Types of Evaluation

Ongoing

1) *planning*
2) *Implement*

Process Evaluation Within process (formative) evaluation, the program's progress is examined, documented, and analyzed. Weekly or monthly budget, staffing, sales, or infection control reports, produced by the organization's management information system, are examples of process evaluation activities. When an unacceptable variance between what was observed and was expected is identified, corrective managerial action is warranted. The purpose of such action is to get the program "back on track." Process evaluation is conducted from the time the program is implemented to its termination. Adjustments are recommended in either the plan or the implementation processes, given the field experience to date. Your program's management objective usually mandates process evaluation which is often reported in the form of monthly, quarterly, bi-annually, and annual reports.

Subpart of process

Implementation Evaluation Within implementation evaluation, the program's implementation experience is investigated, documented, and analyzed. Implementation evaluation is an element of process evaluation and is conducted once, after the program has been in the field for about one-quarter to one-third of its projected life span.

First implementing.

Impact Evaluation Within impact (summative) evaluation, both the intended and unintended final effect(s) of the program are researched, recorded and analyzed. This type of study is conducted either as the program ends or after it terminates. Impact evaluations tend to be rather labor intensive and comprehensive.

Looking at outcome Results

Evaluation Reports

When a program is evaluated, studies are sequenced as: (a) process starts, (b) implementation, (c) process resumes, and (d) impact. Regardless of the type of program evaluation study being conducted, we should document:

Who

a. Who conducted the examination (include relevant dates, funding sources, and assumptions, if any)?
b. Which objectives were examined?
c. How were data obtained (surveys, interviews, chart audits, etc.)?
d. How were data analyzed and presented?
e. What were the factors which enabled and/or hindered objective attainment? and
f. What suggestions for program improvement or modification were gleaned from the results of the study?

When objective, service target, or activity attainment is to be documented by the presence of a copy of something (e.g., a list), such documentation should be placed within an appendix of the relevant report. Statements regarding goal, objective, service target, and activity attainment which require documentation (e.g., a long data table) should have that documentation reserved to an appendix within the relevant evaluation report. A suggested reporting document format is presented in Chapter 7, as are data collection methods. For more information, see *Evaluation of Health Promotion and Education Programs* by Windsor, Baranowski, Clark, and Cutter (1984).

Role of Management Information System The program's management information system is essential in process, implementation, and impact evaluation efforts as it generates reports that can be used to measure the program's compliance with its plan. It then becomes a manager's decision as to whether or not any observed variance is sufficient to warrant corrective action.

AN OPERATIONS PROGRAM EVALUATION MODEL

It is hoped that the above discussion has been sufficient to lay a conceptual foundation for our discussion of the following model. This evaluation model has been designed to assist operations oriented program planners and managers, without an extensive background in evaluation, to evaluate their programs. As structured, the model will facilitate process, implementation, and impact evaluation.

Model Assumptions

This evaluation model rests upon these assumptions:

[handwritten: accomplish objective / you have a goal]

a. The accomplishment of objectives leads to goal attainment;
b. The accomplishment of related service targets and activities leads to objective attainment;
c. Indicators can be developed and specified that render evidence of objective, activity, and service target attainment;
d. The planner and/or program manager has a sufficiently detailed knowledge of the appropriate health specialty to identify or develop and specify indicators; *[handwritten: Detailed]*
e. Management, process, and outcome objectives [or permitted substitutes] have been developed according to strict definition requirements; and *[handwritten: Knowledge]*
f. Available or anticipated resources are sufficient to support program objectives.

Once each of these assumptions has been met, the planner is ready to plot objectives, service targets, and activities on an evaluation grid.

Program Evaluation Grid

The evaluation grid (adapted from Reinke, 1988, pp. 206–208) is a device that requires a program planner or manager to explicitly identify (a) what are program objectives, service targets, and activities; (b) indicators of attainment; and (c) how those indicator data will be obtained and documented. The use of the program evaluation grid enables the planner or manager to determine: (a) degree of objective attainment, (b) whether or not the plan is being implemented as scheduled, and (c) degree of program impact.

Case: Hardee Cog Company, Inc.

Employee Wellness Program Evaluation Grid

Program Goal: To increase the percentage of employees who always wear seatbelts from 12% to 75%, with seatbelt preventable injuries halved by 15 October 1993. (Could substitute as an outcome objective.)

Program Objectives:	Attainment Indicator	Method of Data Gathering
1) To mandate the use of seatbelts 100% of the time by occupants riding or driving in company owned or rented vehicles effective 1 February 1993. (Process Objective)	Company Policy	Company Policy Manual Copy
a) Propose that the president mandate a company-wide seatbelt use policy with a non-compliance sanction by 10 January 1993.	Policy Proposal	Copy of Policy Proposal
b) Testify before the Corporate Executive Committee as to the advantages of such a policy at the 15 January 1993 meeting.	Give Testimony	Copy of testimony in Council minutes
c) Once the policy has been adopted, disseminate the policy to employees through payroll distribution by 25 January 1993.	Copy of Policy to each employee	Each employee receives the policy in his/her check envelope
2) To have 90% of employees attend a seatbelt education session and score at least 75% of correct answers on a quiz by 1 September 1993. (Process Objective)	Computation of attendees over # of employees	Attendance sheets signed at end of session
a) Develop an educational curriculum to educate employees about the advantages of seatbelt use by 1 March 1993.	Curriculum	Copy of curriculum
b) Schedule, advertise, and initiate education sessions (advise supervisors to count as time worked session attendance) from 1 April to 1 September 1993.	Marketing Plan & statement that activity completed	Copy of schedule, sign in sheets, & supervisor memo
c) Conduct 20 educational sessions (20 sessions with an average of 40 participants) by 1 September 1993.	# of sessions held & average # of participants	Report of sessions being held and participant count
d) Conduct ten free educational sessions for employee families and interested community members by 1 September 1993.	# of sessions held	Report of sessions being held

Program Objectives:	Attainment Indicator	Method of Data Gathering
3) To have 90% of employees report positive attitudes towards seatbelt use on a written survey instrument by 30 September 1993. (Process Objective)	Survey results report with supportive data	Copy of report
a) Post five different seatbelt use posters, monthly, in each of ten departments starting in November 1992 for 12 months.	Statement of attainment	Written statement supported by observation
b) Distribute a reminder with each employee pay check between 1 January and 31 October 1993.	Statement of attainment	Copies of 20 reminders
c) Publish the names of employees who are found wearing seatbelts in company vehicles, thus making them eligible for periodic drawings for free gifts to be conducted quarterly between 1 January and 31 October 1993.	Statement of attainment	Copies of the names of contest winners and prize description
d) Operate a free seatbelt information table, using educational literature, between 1 January and 31 October 1993.	Statement of inventory distributed	Depleted stock and copy of inventory
e) Distribute free bumper stickers to employees, and make employees who display the sticker eligible for cash prizes to be awarded quarterly between 1 January and 31 October 1993.	Inventory Statement and statement of attainment	Copy of statement and list of winners and money won
f) Conduct an employee survey to ascertain and report employee attitudes and behaviors concerning seatbelt use by 30 September 1993.	Completed report	Copy of report
4) To efficiently and effectively manage the company's project between 1 November 1992 and 31 October 1993. (Management Objective)	Statement of attainment	Report of project attaining objectives on budget
a) Report to the Executive Committee quarterly between 1 November 1992 and 31 October 1993.	Statement of attainment	Copies of quarterly reports

Program Objectives:	Attainment Indicator	Method of Data Gathering
b) Employ staff by 31 December 1992.	Statement of attainment	Signed contracts
c) Report impact evaluation results by 31 October 1993.	Statement of attainment	Copy of report
d) Design, conduct, and report comprehensive needs analysis addressing employee wellness and disease prevention needs by 31 October 1993.	Completed report	Copy of a report

It is suggested that planners first develop the statement of program goal(s), objectives, service targets, and activities. Second, the program's evaluation grid should be developed. (Make sure that there is a logical relationship between each objective, service target, and activity and the corresponding indicator(s). Additionally, be sure that indicator data can be accurately, efficiently, and legally obtained.) Third, the actual planning document narrative is drafted after the evaluation grid is completed.

The statement of attainment is a declarative statement that the objective, service target, or activity has been met. The health program manager or other designated person(s) should be the only ones given the authority to make such a statement. There should be sufficient "back-up" evidence to support such a claim.

SELECTED ISSUES IN EVALUATION

Ethics

Evaluators should be honest, knowledgeable, and well qualified in their field. It is essential that those relying on an evaluation report have confidence in the results and the principal investigator. Every possible step should be taken to protect the confidentiality of patient records and the identity of those being interviewed. Findings should be stated clearly with supporting documentation. Under no circumstances is it ever acceptable to "fudge" or misrepresent data. Of course, there will be differences over interpretation; but data should be as "clean" as possible. Make every effort to render your best judgments and recommendations, based on data and experience, irrespective of how it may be received.

Objectives Requiring Specialized Knowledge

The objectives, service targets, and activities presented within the Hardee Cog Company example were fairly simple; where specialized knowledge was required, a consultant was to be employed. Program objectives which require the use of quasi-experimental or experimental health service research, epidemiological, or evaluation designs (or statistics or computer programming) should be performed by someone who is specifically trained in those areas. If such personnel are not internally available to the program planning or management team, either find them or hire them.

The retention of consultants is routine and very desirable when the program does not have access to needed specialized knowledge. The following guidelines may be helpful when employing a consultant:

a. Document what the consultant is to do along with specific duties, product descriptions, final report organization, time lines, and method of payment (This document becomes the basis for the preparation of proposals by prospective vendors.);

b. Accept bids from at least 3 consultants, if possible;

c. When negotiating with prospective vendors, know what may be negotiated;

d. Remember, a consultant may not be able to do what is needed for the funds available (If this happens, objective, service target, or activity revision may be necessary. There is nothing wrong with revising a plan, just have a reason.);

e. Have the prospective vendor provide evidence of past successful performance and references;

f. When the product is delivered, pay what was agreed upon (Some consultants will want interval billing, which means that as parts of the product are completed, payment is made. This is fair; but you should decide whether you want to trust the consultant to deliver the final product.); and

g. Include a "zipper clause" which states that everything not expressly stated in the contract is subject to negotiation.

The most important thing to remember is that if you or the planning team lacks the specialized knowledge to accomplish a program objective, either retain a consultant or revise the objective. It should be noted that some consultants will work for free or very reduced fees, depending on the project. Securing the services of one of these nice people will still require the equivalent of a contract, but could perhaps be called a "memorandum of understanding."

Your local higher education institution or professional association are good places to start looking for consultants. The best place to start looking is within your own institution.

SUMMARY

Programs should be evaluated as implemented, after becoming fully operational, and after or during termination. Through evaluation, one learns what worked, what did not, and why. Further, information gained through evaluation is used to improve decision-making. Where specialized knowledge is needed, a consultant should be retained. Whenever a consultant is used, a contract or memorandum of understanding should be employed.

REVIEW QUESTIONS _____

1. A type of research which is designed to produce timely information for use in making judgments concerning program improvement, management, and continuation is:
   a. Epidemiologic
   b. Demographic
   c. Financial
   d. Evaluative

2. The most important difference between health services and evaluation research is:
   a. Differences in types of data utilized
   b. Differences in types of methodologies utilized
   c. Differences in data reporting techniques
   d. Differences in use of judgment concerning programs

3. The type of evaluation study which is conducted as a program ends is:
   a. Process
   b. Implementation
   c. Impact
   d. None of the above

4. When conducting the evaluation of a program, what is the suggested sequence of studies?
   a. Implementation, process, impact
   b. Impact, implementation, impact, process
   c. Process, impact, implementation, process
   d. Process, implementation, process, impact

5. It is suggested that *planners first develop* which one of the following:
   a. Program's evaluation grid
   b. Statement of objectives, etc. goals, services, torgalv
   c. Actual planning document itself
   d. Really doesn't make any difference

6. Which one of the following pairs is incorrect?
   a. Process and formative evaluation are equivalent.
   b. Impact and summative evaluation are equivalent.
   c. Implementation evaluation is an element of impact evaluation.
   d. Implementation evaluation is an element of process evaluation.

7. The type of evaluation where the program is monitored from implementation to termination is called?
   a. Implementation   c. Impact   *Formative*
   b. Process *(Formative)* d. None of the above   *Process*

8. The mandate for process evaluation usually comes from the _____ objective.
   a. Outcome   c. Management
   b. Process   d. Summative

9. When is it considered most appropriate to employ a consultant?
   a. When there is money in the budget for one
   b. When the planner lacks specialized knowledge   /
   c. When the planner has too much work to do
   d. When the manager's sister needs a job

10. What is the suggested sequence in developing the planning document?
   a. Goal and objective statement, the narrative, then the evaluation grid
   b. The evaluation grid, the narrative, then the goal and objective statement
   c. The narrative, goal and objective statement, then the evaluation grid
   d. The goal and objective statement, the evaluation grid, then the narrative

DISCUSSION QUESTIONS _____

1. What are some common characteristics of evaluation?

2. Explain how process and impact evaluation are related to each other and how they are different.

3. Describe how you would evaluate an objective which requires knowledge you do not have. Also, describe some considerations you might take into account.
   I would not   Consultant

4. For the goal and supporting objectives, service targets, and activities developed for discussion question 5 in chapter 2, construct an evaluation grid.

4

A Planning Documentation Model

Chapter Objective:

1. Describe the health planning documentation model.

As mentioned earlier, there are many different models for writing health planning documents. Your institution may have a required format. Most of the requests for proposals (RFPs) announced by funding agencies have a required format which must be followed including page limitations. Irrespective of the required document format, each one contains essentially the same information. The model proposed here is based on what has been discussed within the previous three chapters. The model is presented below.

MODEL FOR WRITING A HEALTH PLANNING DOCUMENT

The model consists of four sections: (a) program/project description, (b) budget description, (c) appendices, and (d) references. As recommended, the program's mission, goal(s), objectives, service targets, activities, and evaluation grid have already been composed; it is also a good idea to have already developed the program's budget. These then become the basis for completing the rest of the health planning document. Following is a summary of each section (with an explanation of desirable content) presented in a sequential format.

I. *Project Description*
   Each section should be written in paragraph form with complete sentences and with each page numbered.
   A. *Statement of the Problem:* Presented within this section is text which describes the problem to be addressed by the proposed project. Include, as appropriate, a description of the target population, relevant indicator data, anticipated conse-

quences if intervention does not occur, and other relevant data which *describe the problem*. This section may be a few paragraphs in length.

B. *Project Justification:* Described within this section is why THIS PARTICULAR project is needed. Discuss any potential benefits of intervening into the problem as a result of this particular project. *The potential benefit(s) of the project should be similar to its stated goal(s) which in turn must be directed to solving the problem described in Section I.A.* Such benefits could include increased market share, departmental efficiency, departmental effectiveness, risk aversion, or financial rewards. If detailed supporting documentation is needed, reserve such to an appendix; but be sure to include the appendix letter and/or title in this section. This section may be a few paragraphs or a few pages in length.

C. *Summary of Project Methodology:* Within this section is described how the proposed project intends to achieve stated goal(s). Avoid repeating the program's objectives, service targets, and activities word-for-word. Instead *summarize, in general terms, what type of actions the plan's objectives require in order to achieve the goal(s). (Draw on each objective's service targets and/or activities for this discussion.)* This section may consist of a few paragraphs or pages.

D. *Summary of Expected Outcomes:* Again, don't repeat the program's goal or objectives word-for-word. *Restate the major benefit and related minor benefits of the program* as briefly as possible. Be sure to document that the problem described in Section A will be at least reduced (better if eliminated) when the plan is fully implemented. *Make sure that your methodology will support what you claim.*

E. *Evaluation Element:* Presented within this section is a description of how the project proposes to manage services and evaluate impact. This requires data. *Thus, contained within this section is a description of the indicator data that will be used to establish whether or not the program's goal(s) and objectives (process and outcome) have been achieved. This section also describes how such data will be collected, tabulated, analyzed, reported, and used.*

Make reference to the evaluation grid, which may have been reserved to an appendix. (If you think the program's chances of acceptance will be increased if the evaluation grid is included within the body of this section, include it.)

Describe what (and when) evaluation studies will be conducted. Be sure to make reference to the management information system that will be used to support plan evaluation activities. Refer to the proposed program's Gantt Chart, which should be included within this section or reserved to an appendix. Label the Gantt Chart as a figure and include it on its own page, even if the Gantt Chart is reserved to an appendix.

If an objective requires a consultant to evaluate attainment, so state and refer the reader to an appendix which contains the consultant's resume if one has already been identified. It may be necessary to have a consultant help prepare this section. Most will do so at no cost in the anticipation of a consulting contract. This section will vary in length from a few paragraphs to a few pages.

F. *Marketing Element:* Most programs/projects probably will have a marketing element. Such elements may have internal components (within the institution) or external (outside the institution) components. *Describe within this section how people will be made aware of the proposed program or project.* For example, one might cite that posters, payroll stuffers, or ads will be used. Do not include how you intend to gain plan acceptance in this section. If your program or proposal doesn't need a marketing element, don't write one. Guidelines for preparing a marketing plan are found in Chapter Nine.

II. *Budget Description*

This section consists of two sub-components: (a) budget, usually line item and (b) budget justification statement, which *briefly* describes the rationale for each line item category. Detailed explanations are reserved to an appendix which is cited in the line item's justification. If a line item presented in this model is excluded from a program budget, omit the line.

A. *Personnel: Personnel positions are named, as are their cost in terms of salary* (hourly or yearly) *and fringe benefits.* In this section refer to position descriptions which are reserved to an appendix. (Such descriptions can be batched or each description can be placed in a separate appendix.) If staff have already been identified and the chances of program acceptance will be improved, include their resumes, each in its own appendix.

B. *Travel:* Travel costs are presented by position. Included in determining travel costs are mileage, per diem, common carrier fares, and meals.

C. *Office Support:* Office support costs include office equipment, furniture, supplies, space, utilities, and telephone equipment and lines.

D. *Educational Materials:* Educational materials can include both equipment (e.g., film projector or VCR) and/or printed materials (e.g., books or pamphlets). If detailed data explaining the cost and rationale for materials selection is necessary, reserve to an appendix. Be sure to cite the appendix in the budget justification section. If the proposed program does not require such materials, omit this line item.

E. *Clinical Materials:* Clinical materials can include both the cost of medical, dental, or laboratory equipment and/or necessary supplies. Reserve detailed explanations to an appendix. If the proposed program does not require clinical materials, omit this line item.

F. *Continuing Education:* The cost of providing continuing education for program staff is presented in this section.

G. *Other Costs:* Miscellaneous costs are presented within this section and may include catering, speaker honorariums, or marketing costs. If allowable, indirect costs may be included in this section.

III. Appendices

The number of appendices and the size of each appendix varies greatly. Irrespective of the number, each appendix is to be labeled with a letter and title. Each appendix is to be page numbered. Each appendix is to appear in the order it is cited in the text of the proposal.

IV. References

All references cited within the text or an appendix are to be listed in this section of the document. References take the form of professional trade journals, research journals, interviews, price quotes, business communications, internal management reports, or related sources of information that contribute to the development of the program/project plan. It is unacceptable to fail to report references.

Remember, it is important to link goals and objectives explicitly in a planning document. Explicit linkage will increase a reviewer's confidence in the planner's or manager's ability to accomplish stated goal(s) and objectives. Be detailed enough in the planning document, so that in a few months, you will recall exactly what was proposed. Be sure to determine whether or not your institution has policies, procedures, and/or rules concerning indirect costs, internal review processes, or any matter pertaining to the planning, implementation, and operation of the planned program. If the plan is funded or approved, you will be obliged to complete it. Be as realistic as possible.

Your documentation objective is to inform and impress. Accordingly, the planning document should be concise, lucid, easy to read, and grammatically correct. Reference citations should be recorded consistently. It is a good idea to use a style manual. By following the outline presented below, you will help ensure that the document is presentable:

a. Edit the document for content and logic. Have at least two other knowledgeable peers edit the document.

b. Proofread the document for visual layout; grammer, spelling, and punctuation; and style, flow, and fit. After major editing, proofread the document again.

c. Have your proofreading and editing tools available. These tools include: (a) a recent, comprehensive dictionary, (b) a thesaurus, and (c) a style manual. Use your wordprocessing program's spell-checker.

d. Determine the time when proofreading and editing are best performed. Proofread and edit only during that time. Proofread and edit in an environment that is comfortable. Remember, what is desired is accuracy—not speed.

The appearance of the planning document makes a statement in the reader's mind about the quality of the plan and the competence of the planner. The planning document is an opportunity to make a clear, positive statement about the plan and yourself. These aforementioned suggestions apply to documents prepared for virtually all purposes.

Please refer to Appendix 4.A for a sample health plan for Hardee Cog Company's Wellness Program which is based on the above model. Presented within Appendix 4.B is a sample proposal reviewer evaluation form.

SUMMARY

All health plans should be documented. Documentation models typically include a program or project description, budget justification, appendices, and references. The document should be well-written, grammatically correct, accurately punctuated, and words correctly spelled. A plan's documentation plants an image in a reader's mind about the quality of the plan and the competence of the planner.

Appendix 4.A

The Hardee Cog Company
Employee Wellness Program Proposal

Title: Hardee Cog Company Employee Wellness Program

Submitted By: William Hardee, Chair
Employee Wellness Planning Group

Budget Requested: $49,939.30

Submission Date: 1 December 1992

I. PROJECT DESCRIPTION

Statement of the Problem

Within the past 16 months the Hardee Cog Company has experienced 3 deaths and 18 known injuries resulting in the loss of productive manhours and increased claims costs of $275,000.00 for the company's self-insurance program. Two of the 18 injured have retired on disability; 12 have returned to work after consuming an average of 175 sick leave hours, costing the company an estimated $15,750.00; and 4 remain off work.[1]

These deaths and injuries probably could have been prevented had those employees and family members been wearing seatbelts. Data from the recent behavioral risk factor prevalence survey indicated that 67 percent (n = 530) of employees do not routinely wear seatbelts.[2] Information concerning the seatbelt use of family members is not available.

As a corporate family, Hardee Cog Company has lost valuable members to death and injury as well as much income to preventable accidents. Such conditions are expected to continue to prevail unless intervention is undertaken.

Project Justification

The proposed program will create a corporate environment where seatbelt use is encouraged and supported by sympathetic employee attitudes, corporate policy, and the corporate mission:

"The corporate mission of Hardee Cog is to produce a high quality cog and to make a positive contribution to the welfare of our customers, employees, and home community"[3]

As a result of the program, the premature death, disability, and injury related to the lack or inconsistent use of seatbelts will be reduced, thereby reducing the cost of human suffering and financial drain to the company. It is projected that by 15 October 1993, 75 percent of company employees will report "always" wearing seatbelts, and that seatbelt preventable injuries will be halved to no more than nine, with zero fatalities.

Project Methodology

The program will advocate for a mandated company policy which requires the use of seatbelts at all times while driving or riding in company owned or rented vehicles. The placing of 5 different posters in each department monthly; operating a free literature table; distributing reminders each pay day; and providing free bumper stickers which makes an employee eligible for cash and prizes will help create a supportive environment for seatbelt use.

Professional staff of the proposed program will research, design, implement, and instructionally evaluate a seatbelt education curriculum which addresses the unique needs and concerns of the Hardee Cog Company corporate family. By offering 20 educational sessions to employees and 10 to family members, ample opportunity to learn facts relative to seatbelt use and to develop supportive attitudes towards seatbelt use will be available. Instructional activities will be designed to provide needed information and to assist the participant to develop supportive attitudes. Professional program staff will be available to individually answer employee and family member questions and to address concerns. Attendance by employees at educational sessions will be strongly encouraged, but not required. Attendance at employee educational sessions will be counted as time worked and not charged to the proposed program. By 30 September 1993, employees will be surveyed as to seatbelt use and attitudes as well as other behavioral health risk prevalence, wellness program needs, and desired programs.

Expected Outcomes

It is expected that, as a result of the proposed program, at least 75 percent of employees will always use seatbelts when driving or riding in a vehicle. Further, at least 90 percent of employees will report supportive seatbelt use attitudes. Preventable death and disability will be lessened and the number of injuries will be halved, thus contributing to a safe, healthful, and productive work environment. Also, safe behaviors, learned on the job by company employees, will transfer to their homes and families.

Evaluation Element

Presented in Sub-Appendix A is the program's evaluation grid, which presents each program objective, service target, and activity along with the indicator(s) which will signify attainment as well as how such data will be obtained. Records of attendance, copies of documents, survey result reports, depleted stocks of educational materials, and quarterly reports by program staff will be used to evaluate goal, objective, and service target attainment. An implementation evaluation (April) and impact evaluation (September) will be conducted with reports submitted to the Executive Committee. The instructional efficacy of educational sessions will be evaluated by a quiz at the end of each session. The quiz will be developed during the curriculum writing process. The health education specialist will be responsible for ensuring that the administrative and financial practices of the program are conducted in accordance with Company policy and procedure. The specialist will be responsible for developing the program's management information system to track data related to goal and objective attainment. Data will reside within a database capable of tabulating data into charts, graphs, and/or tables, as needed.

The health education specialist will be responsible for maintaining the quality of educational services in accordance with acceptable standards of practice. The specialist will conduct needed employee surveys, including a comprehensive needs analysis which is to be completed by October.

The program's management objective requires continuous monitoring and quarterly reporting. The development of the program's management information system and regular staff meetings ensure objective attainment. A Gantt chart has been developed to facilitate project management. (See Sub-Appendix B.)

Marketing Element

Program services and contests will be marketed via the employee newpaper, posters, and announcements at staff meetings. Program staff will attend employee staff meetings to describe the program. Professional staff will be available for individual conferences.

II. Budget Description

HARDEE COG COMPANY EMPLOYEE WELLNESS PROGRAM BUDGET

	Amount	**Total**
Personnel-Positions		$33,000.00
Health Education Specialist	$25,000.00	
Secretary	8,000.00	
Personnel-Fringe Benefits		9,639.30
Health Education Specialist	7,302.50	
Secretary	2,336.80	
Travel		1,000.00
Office Support		3,100.00
Office Equipment	2,500.00	
Office Supplies	600.00	
Educational Materials		1,300.00
Instructional Equipment	1,000.00	
Printed Materials	300.00	
Continuing Education		300.00
Other Costs		1,600.00
Cash Awards	800.00	
Prizes	800.00	
	Total =	$49,939.30

BUDGET JUSTIFICATION STATEMENT

Personnel-Positions

One full-time equivalent (FTE) position is needed: Health Education Specialist. A one-half time secretary is needed. See Sub-Appendix C for position descriptions. Positions are funded for ten months. Such a staffing pattern is needed to effect program goal, objective, and service target attainment.

Personnel-Fringe Benefits

Using Hardee Cog Company's standard fringe benefit rate of 29.21 percent of salary, the cost of program employee fringe benefits is $9,639.30. Such a fringe benefit package is needed to attract and retain high quality personnel.

Travel

Travel is projected to cost $1,000.00, which includes mileage, per diem, meals (standard company rates), and travel costs to a national meeting for the health eudcation specialist.

Office Support

There are no office space, furniture, or utilities costs charged to the project. There are two vacant offices (with furniture) in the Employee Health Section of the Human Resources Department. Office equipment (computer bundle, printer, and typewriter) costs are projected to be $2,500.00. Computer software programs are available at no cost to the program. Office supply costs are projected to be $600.00. Telephone equipment, service, and lines are available to the program at no charge. These materials are needed to support the program.

Educational Materials

The projected costs of instructional equipment is $1000.00 (flip chart [and 3 refills] and stand, VCR with monitor and stand, and seatbelt education video). Printed materials (pamphlets, posters, printed bumper stickers) are projected to cost $300.00. The materials are essential to accomplish educational objectives.

Continuing Education

For professional employees, the company allows $300.00 yearly for continuing education reimbursement. For the specialist, $300.00 is requested.

Other Costs

As the proposed program is operational for eight months, award and prize costs are $1,600.00 (8-$100 awards and 16-$50 prizes).

Appendix 4.A

Sub-Appendix A
Program Evaluation Grid

Program Goal: To increase the percentage of employees who always wear seatbelts from 12% to 75%, with seatbelt preventable injuries halved by 15 October 1993.

Program Objectives:	Attainment Indicator	Method of Data Gathering
1) To mandate the use of seatbelts 100% of the time by occupants riding or driving in company owned or rented vehicles effective 1 February 1993.	Company policy	Company policy manual copy
a) Propose that the president mandate a company-wide seatbelt use policy with a non-compliance sanction by 10 January 1993.	Policy proposal	Copy of policy proposal
b) Testify before the Corporate Executive Committee as to the advantages of such a policy at the 15 January 1993 meeting.	Give testimony	Copy of testimony in council minutes
c) Once the policy has been adopted, disseminate the policy to employees through payroll distribution by 25 January 1993.	Copy of policy to each employee	Each employee receives his check envelope
2) To have 90% of employees attend a seatbelt education session and score at least 75% of correct answers on a quiz by 1 September 1993.	Computation of attendees over # of employees	Attendance sheets signed at end of session
a) Develop an educational curriculum to educate employees about the advantages of seatbelt use by 1 March 1993.	Curriculum	Copy of curriculum

Program Objectives:	Attainment Indicator	Method of Data Gathering
b) Schedule, advertise, and initiate education sessions (advise supervisors to count as time worked session attendance) from 1 April to 1 September 1993.	Marketing plan & completed activity statement	Copy of schedule, sign-in sheets, & supervisor memo
c) Conduct 20 educational sessions (20 sessions with an average of 40 participants) by 1 September 1993.	# of sessions held & average # of participants	Report of sessions being held and participant count
d) Conduct 10 free educational sessions for employee families and interested community members by 1 September 1993.	# of sessions held	Report of sessions being held
3) To have 90% of employees report positive attitudes towards seatbelt use on a written survey instrument by 30 September 1993.	Survey results report with supportive data	Copy of report
a) Post five different seatbelt use posters monthly for 12 months in each of ten departments starting in November 1992.	Statement of attainment	Written statement supported by observation
b) Distribute a reminder with each employee pay check between 1 January and 31 October 1993.	Statement of attainment	Copies of 20 reminders
c) Publish the names of employees who are found wearing seatbelts in company vehicles, thus making them eligible for periodic drawings for free gifts to be conducted quarterly between 1 January and 31 October 1993.	Statement of attainment	Copies of the names of contest winners and prize description

Program Objectives:	Attainment Indicator	Method of Data Gathering
d) Operate a free seatbelt information table using educational literature between 1 January and 31 October 1993.	Statement of inventory distributed	Depleted stock and copy of inventory
e) Distribute free bumper stickers to employees and make employees who display the sticker eligible for cash prizes to be awarded quarterly between 1 January and 31 October 1993.	Inventory statement and statement of attainment	Copy of statement and list of winners and money won
f) Conduct employee survey to ascertain and report employee attitudes and behaviors concerning seatbelt use by 30 September 1993.	Completed report	Survey
4) To efficiently and effectively manage the company's project between 1 November 1992 and 31 October 1993.	Statement of attainment	Report of project attaining objectives on budget
a) Report to the Executive Committee quarterly between 1 November 1992 and 31 October 1993.	Statement of attainment	Quarterly reports
b) Employ staff by 31 December 1992.	Statement of attainment	Signed contracts
c) Report implementation evaluation results by 1 March 1993.	Statement of attainment	Copy of report
d) Report impact evaluation results by 31 October 1993.	Statement of attainment	Copy of report
e) Design, conduct and report a comprehensive needs analysis addressing employee wellness and disease prevention needs by 31 October 1993.	Completed report	Copy of report

Appendix 4.A

Sub-Appendix B
Program Management Gantt Chart

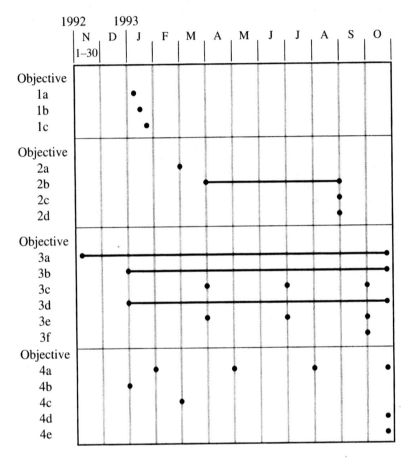

Figure 4.1   Program Management Gantt Chart

Appendix 4.A

Sub-Appendix C
Position Descriptions

Position: **Health Education Specialist**

Education: A Masters Degree in Health Education or Adult Education (with health background). Preference will be given to a nationally certified health education specialist.

Experience:	At least 3 years experience in the design and delivery of corporate wellness programs and some program management experience.
Duties:	Develop educational curricula
	Conduct educational sessions
	Select educational equipment
	Select educational materials
	Design educational printed materials
	Design program promotional materials
	Develop wellness program proposals
	Develop project MIS
	Prepare management reports
	Conduct instructional and program evaluation studies
	Design and conduct surveys
	Must be computer literature
	Perform other duties as assigned
Position:	**Secretary**
Education:	An Associate Degree in Secretarial Sciences or 5 years comprehensive experience.
Experience:	2 years experience with the AS Degree or 5 years experience. Must be proficient in wordprocessing, database management, and spreadsheet applications.
Duties:	Maintain program database and electronic spread sheet
	Wordprocess as required
	Maintain program files
	Order supplies and materials as required
	Answer telephones and direct calls
	Engage in general secretarial support services

REFERENCES

[1]Human Resources Department, Employee Health Section Fiscal Year (October, 1991 to September, 1992) Report.

[2]Human Resources Department, Employee Health Section Behavioral Health Risk Prevalence Survey Report, 1992.

[3]Corporate Mission Statement, Adopted 3 October 1972.

Appendix 4.B

Proposal Reviewer Evaluation Form

Health planning documents which are used as proposals are typically reviewed by experts and rated. Often, it is this rating which determines which proposals are funded and which are not. Following is a sample reviewer rating sheet.

Proposals will be rated on a scale of zero to 100. Proposals receiving the highest rating will be funded. Study each proposal carefully and then rate each according to the following criteria. The range for each of the ten criteria is from zero to 10. Total points are then added to arrive at the overall rating.

1. The proposal's goal is consistent with the organization's mission. _____

2. The proposal's objectives are consistent with its goal and the organization's mission. _____

3. The proposal's service targets and activities are consistent with and supportive of its objectives. _____

4. The proposal's attainment indicators are reliable as a means of assessing objective, service target, and activity attainment. _____

5. The proposal's means of indicator verification is both reasonable and possible. _____

6. The proposal's methodology is consistent with and supportive of its objectives. _____

7. The proposal's staffing plan is consistent with and supportive of its objectives. _____

8. The proposal's expected outcomes (i.e., objectives) are sufficiently supported by its budget. _____

9. The proposal's internal and/or external marketing sufficiently supports its objectives. _____

10. The proposal's time frame is realistic given its objectives, service targets, and activities. _____

Total Points _____

SECTION *II*

Health Planning Methods

5

Health Planning Methods: Demography

Chapter Objectives:

1. Describe demographic variables commonly used in health planning.
2. Read and interpret demographic data commonly used in health planning.

It is impossible to plan most health programs or projects in the absence of data. Data, when interpreted, provide the planner with the information necessary to conceive a useful, reliable plan. Therefore, it is essential for any planner or program manager to have as much pertinent, reliable data available for planning as possible.

This chapter will consider the following: (a) the use of demography in health planning and (b) selected issues regarding the use of demography in health planning. The intent is to acquaint you with the descriptive application of demography in operations health planning activities. Reference will be made to other sources of information as warranted.

Demographic data are essential to (a) describe a population's age, race, gender, or other characteristics and (b) describe health services utilization or some other event or behavior of interest, so as to plan and/or target health programs and resources to those most in need or at greatest risk. Both uses of demographic data, as applied to health planning, will be examined.

POPULATION DESCRIPTION

Demographic data include those data which describe a population or target group in terms of such characteristics as age, gender, race or ethnic origin, income, occupation, marital status, or other relevant characteristics.

In 1985, a behavioral risk factor telephone survey of Collier County, Florida adults was conducted by the Collier County Health Department. In order to ascertain how closely the sample reflected true population parameters (i.e., characteristics), a comparison between sample demographic values and the findings from the 1980 US Census of Collier County adults was made. With respect to age and race, the sample characteristics approximated the population parameters (Table 5.1). However, the sample was better educated and wealthier than the population from which it was drawn. Males were undersampled.

To control for the variance between the sample and the population, these data were statistically weighted in order to enable sample characteristics to correspond to population parameters. If these data had not been weighted, then what was found as a result of the study might not be accurate when the health behaviors of persons of various educational levels, gender, and income groupings were examined.

If you are going to do your own study, you will need to decide what demographic variables to include. A useful rule is to clearly define the study's purpose and the intended use for those data which are collected. Once this has been done, select those demographic variables that best meet the study's purpose and intended uses.

Table 5.1 Demographic characteristics of Collier County, Florida adults by 1980 US Census and 1985 sample

Characteristic	Percent		Characteristic	Percent	
	Census	Sample		Census	Sample
Age			*Education*		
18–24	12.0	9.5	<8th grade	14.9	4.8
25–34	16.5	18.5	9–12 years	13.9	12.6
35–44	13.0	13.9	High. Sch. Grad.	35.5	28.9
45–54	12.9	10.5	Some College	17.2	23.5
55–64	19.4	19.2	College Grad.	11.2	21.5
65+	26.0	28.1	Post Grad. Work	7.2	8.2
Race			*Gender*		
White	95.3	95.3	Male	48.5	37.9
Nonwhite	4.7	4.7	Female	51.5	62.1
		Income			
<$14,999	44.9	24.3	25–34,999	12.5	12.9
15–24,999	25.9	27.3	35,000+	16.7	24.1
			Unknown		11.4

Source: Hale, C.D. (1986). *1985 Behavioral Health Risks of Collier County, Florida Adults.* Naples: Collier County Public Health Department.

HEALTH SERVICES UTILIZATION DESCRIPTION _____

Introduction

A second application of demography in health planning is to describe health services utilization or some other event or behavior of interest. It is through such description that health planners are able to describe and, in many instances, explain or predict health services utilization.

Applications demographic data in this manner include: (a) the identification of patterns or trends that might guide decision-making regarding resource allocation or the targeting of intervention efforts, (b) the formulation of goals and/or objectives, (c) the prioritization of interventions, given resource limitations, to those at greatest risk or in most need, and (d) the generation of baseline data, so as to have a comparison group against which to contrast post-intervention results. When demographic data are utilized in these ways, they are merged with non-demographic data, such as those presented in Table 5.3, thus yielding very useful information for use in health planning.

A Model for Ordering Demographic Variables

Since there are a number of demographic variables, it may be helpful to group them in order to facilitate use in health planning, such as in data interpretation. Aday and Shortell (1988, pp. 65–72) have developed a convenient model for ordering (i.e., grouping) demographic variables. Please refer to Table 5.2.

Predisposing variables are those which affect the need to utilize health services. Enabling variables are those which increase the likelihood of health service utilization. Need variables are those related to a need for health services utilization as defined by a patient or a health service provider. A discussion follows.

Table 5.2 The Aday and Shortell model for describing health services utilization by demographic variables

Variables:		
Predisposing	**Enabling**	**Need**
Age	Income	Perceived
Gender	Residence	Evaluated
Race		
Ethnicity		
Education		

Predisposing: Age The age structure of a population has a significant influence upon its health needs and behaviors. The young and the old consume the largest proportion of US health services, hence, they account for significant costs. When planning health services for the young and/or the old, recognize that service level, service intensity, manpower, and costs will most certainly be higher for these groups. This is to be expected as persons in these groups are more likely to be dependent upon society or family members and in greatest need.

Predisposing: Gender Gender is related to health services utilization. Females tend to utilize health services more than males, especially during the reproductive years. Females tend to have higher hospital discharge rates (Graves, 1991, p. 2) and health services utilization than males (DeLozier and Gagnon, 1991, p. 3).

Predisposing: Race Race is also associated with health services utilization. In 1989, whites utilized health services more than blacks or any other racial group (DeLozier and Gagnon, 1991, p. 3). Whites were more likely to have a usual source of health care than blacks, 83 to 77.1 percent (Cornelius, Beauregard and Cohen, 1991, p. 4). Between 1984 and 1988, blacks made fewer physician visits than whites, 4.6 versus 5.4 visits per person, per year (Ries and Brown, 1991, p. 7). Blacks were less likely to have health insurance coverage in 1989 than whites, 20.2 as compared to 12.8 percent (Ries, 1991, p. 2).

Predisposing: Ethnicity Health services utilization differs from ethnic group to ethnic group. For example, 39 percent of Hispanic mothers received no prenatal care during the first trimester as compared to 21 percent of non-Hispanic whites (National Center for Health Statistics, 1990). While 83 percent of whites reported a usual source of health care services, only 72.1 percent of Hispanic Americans claimed a usual source of care in 1987 (Cornelius, Beauregard and Cohen, 1991, p. 8). Hispanic Americans and blacks were less likely to receive ambulatory care in a physician's office than whites (Cornelius, Beauregard and Cohen, 1991, p. 9).

Predisposing: Education The effect of education varies according to the health services utilization indicator (Aday and Shortell, 1988, p. 70). Ries found a direct relationship between educational attainment and having insurance coverage (1991, p. 2). Aday and Shortell reported that those with higher levels of educational attainment were more likely to utilize preventive health services than those with less education (1988, p. 70). Irizarry (1988) reported that elderly persons with low educational attainment were more likely to need health services than those with higher educational attainment.

Enabling: Income Family income affects health service utilization. Ries (1991, p. 2) reported a direct relationship between family income and health insurance coverage. In 1987, families with high levels of income were more likely to have a regular source of health care than families with lower levels of income (Cornelius, Beauregard and Cohen, 1991, p. 8). The combination of health insurance and a usual source of health care combine to encourage health services utilization. The advent of Medicaid and Medicare have done much to increase the access of poor persons to health care services. Persons with lower income levels made more physician visits (1984–1988) than did those from higher income groups (Ries and Brown, 1991, p. 7).

 Enabling: Residence   Residence is related to health services utilization. Typically, people living in rural areas were less likely to have a usual source of care than those living in urban areas. People living in the Midwest were more likely to have a usual source of health care than those living in the West or the South (Cornelius, Beauregard and Cohen, 1991, p. 8). Persons residing in the Northeast United States utilized inpatient acute care services more than those residing in other regions of the country and had an average longer length of stay (Graves, 1991, p. 2). Persons living in the central city and outside a standard metropolitan statistical area (SMSA) were more likely not to have health insurance (Ries, 1991, p. 2). Persons living outside a SMSA were less likely to visit a physician when experiencing a limitation in physical activity (Ries and Brown, 1991, p. 7).

Need: Perceived   According to Aday and Shortell (1988, p. 71), "need is consistently borne out to be the most important predictor of the use of health services." People who rated their health as poor or fair experienced more restricted-activity days, made more physician visits, and utilized more hospital days than those rating their health as good to excellent (Ries and Brown, 1991, p. 5). Those persons rating their health as poor to fair were more likely to have health insurance than those rating health status as good or excellent (Cornelius, Beauregard and Cohen, 1991, p. 5). Such would be expected as those who perceived their health as poor are more likely to utilize health services, and hence, need insurance to assist with payment.

Need: Evaluated   Aday and Shortell (1988, p. 72) have described evaluated need as "Providers' and patients' evaluations of medical need may not always agree. Indicators of providers' evaluations of patients' conditions include their assessment of the actual severity of presenting symptoms or complaints and diagnosis, based on laboratory tests and clinical judgments." Since physicians and other health care providers make referrals and decisions which lead to health service utilization, their determination of need is very important in understanding utilization behaviors. Also, health policy makers rely on perceptions of evaluated need (or proxy indicators) to allocate health resources. Berk, Cunningham, and Beauregard (1991) concluded that the actual number of poor people in a geographical area, rather than per capita income, was a better criterion to use in allocating health care resources. If this recommendation were to be adopted, health policy makers would be operating on evaluated need, i.e., that the more poor persons in an area, the greater the need for an allocation of health care resources.

A Further Example

By way of another example, let's suppose that we are planning a public information campaign concerning the Human Immunodeficiency Virus (HIV) and Acquired Immunodeficiency Syndrome (AIDS). The campaign is to be targeted towards women. The data presented in Table 5.3 will be useful in developing content and in precisely targeting commercials and public service announcements (PSAs).

The first section of the table presents numerical estimates of the number of married and unmarried women, aged 15–44 years, in the United States by selected race categories. The remaining two sections of the table describe how respondents to the National Survey of Family Growth, which was conducted by the National Center for Health Statistics (NCHS), answered questions concerning HIV/AIDS transmission.

A larger percentage of unmarried (22.1%) than of all women (19.5%) believed that HIV/AIDS can be transmitted by giving a blood donation. When comparing race, about one-third of non-Hispanic black women reported holding that belief across all marital status categories. Concerning HIV/AIDS transmission through being bitten by an infected insect, a larger percentage of unmarried women (24.6%) held that false belief than did married women (21.6%) in 1988. Again, non-Hispanic black women were more likely to report that belief than non-Hispanic white women, across all marital categories.

We could develop and deliver commercials or PSAs designed to educate selected categories of women about HIV transmission via a medium most likely to reach the intended target audience. Further, we could re-administer the survey to evaluate the effectiveness of our public information campaign.

The use of demographic data, in such an application, enables the planner (and/or program manager) to be more precise in targeting interventions and/or resources. This increase in precision helps programs to be more efficient and effective, as well as accountable.

CONSIDERATIONS IN THE USE OF DEMOGRAPHIC DATA

Evaluating Data Quality and Accuracy

When reviewing and considering the use of demographic data, it is a good idea to evaluate the quality and accuracy of those data. This can be done by (a) comparing suspect data findings to what was expected; (b) comparing suspect data to existing data which is known to be of high quality; (c) asking a known expert to evaluate the suspect data; (d) examining the suspect data for consistency within itself; and (e) evaluating the suspect data for compatibility with what is already known. Remember, none of these techniques are foolproof; it is probably best to use a combination of techniques. Also, each method assumes a familiarity with the subject under consideration.

What you believe.

Table 5.3 Number of women 15–44 and percent with misinformation about selected means of HIV/AIDS transmission, 1988

Transmission/ Characteristic	All Women	Marital Status		
		Currently	Formerly	Never
		(Number in Thousands)		
All Women	57,900	29,147	7,695	21,058
Unmarried	28,753	...	7,695	21,058
Race:				
Non-Hispanic white	42,575	23,367	5,212	13,996
Non-Hispanic black	7,408	2,102	1,355	3,951
		Donating Blood (Percent)		
All women	19.5	16.9	21.6	22.3
Unmarried women	22.1	...	21.6	22.3
Race:				
Non-Hispanic white	15.4	13.8	17.5	17.3
Non-Hispanic black	32.1	28.3	31.5	34.4
		Being Bitten by an Infected Insect (Percent)		
All women	21.6	18.6	22.7	25.3
Unmarried women	24.6	...	22.7	25.3
Race:				
Non-Hispanic white	19.2	17.3	19.9	22.1
Non-Hispanic black	29.8	26.9	29.5	31.5

Source: McNally, J. W., Moser, W. D. *AIDS-Related Knowledge and Behavior Among Women 15–44 Years of Age: United States, 1988* (Advance Data no 200.) Hyattsville, MD: National Center for Health Statistics, 1991.

When comparing the results of various studies, be sure to examine the demographics upon which those findings rest. If the demographic characteristics of the samples or populations vary greatly, you might exercise caution when considering whether or not to use those findings in your planning activities. A recent example of this is that some projects funded or conducted by the National Institutes of Health, from which we have learned much about heart disease, cholesterol, and cancer, have systematically excluded women. It is yet unclear as to whether or not this bias has tainted what is known about several significant national health problems.

Sources of Demographic Data

There are several sources of demographic data. The most commonly utilized sources include: (a) the US Census, (b) vital statistics offices and reports [usually available from your local health department], (c) local chambers of commerce, (d) local or state planning agencies, (e) your institutional record system (or those of allied agencies), (f) National Center for Health Statistics, (g) Centers for Disease Control and Prevention, (h) professional or voluntary organizations, (i) the state or federal Bureau of Labor Statistics, (j) journals, and (k) conferences.

SUMMARY

Organizing data by various demographic variables is useful. Such organization helps guide planner's efforts to efficiently and effective target resources. Demographic data may be gathered from a variety of sources. However, all demographic data must be evaluated for quality and accuracy prior to use.

Demographic data are used to describe a population, health services utilization, or some other object of interest. With respect to health services utilization, demographic variables are grouped as either predisposing, enabling, or need related. Predisposing variables include age, gender, race, ethnicity, and education. Enabling variables are income and residence. Need is defined to include both perceived and evaluated conditions.

REVIEW AND APPLICATION QUESTIONS

Directions. Read each question very carefully before selecting your answer. There is one correct answer for each question.

1. Data which only includes population or target group characteristics such as age and gender are:
   - a. Epidemiologic
   - b. Demographic
   - c. Financial
   - d. Evaluative

2. The definition, "variables are those which increase the likelihood of health service utilization," defines:
   - a. Predisposing
   - b. Perceived Need
   - c. Enabling
   - d. Evaluated Need

3. The definition, "variables are those related to health service utilization as defined by a patient," defines:
   - a. Predisposing
   - b. Perceived Need
   - c. Enabling
   - d. Evaluated Need

4. Which type of variable is "residence" considered?
   - a. Predisposing
   - b. Perceived Need
   - c. Enabling
   - d. Evaluated Need

5. Techniques for evaluating the quality and/or accuracy of demographic data include all of the following EXCEPT:
   a. Comparing suspect data to those of known quantity
   b. Comparing suspect data to what was expected
   c. Comparing suspect data to what is already known
   d. Having a known expert review the suspect data

Pg 66

Case 1: Northwest County Health Department

Read the following health services research report and answer the following questions.

The Northwest County Public Health Department commissioned a study of the health care seeking behaviors of county residents (population 33,000). Northwest County (2,000 square miles) is located in the northern reaches of a western state. The region surrounding the county is rural, with the chief businesses being ranching, farming, and lumbering. There is a large retired population. The county seat's population is 10,000. There are three smaller towns in the county, with the largest being 1,200 in population. Per capita income is $11,500, with the average household size being 3.6 persons. You have obtained a summary of the report with the following data:

Table 1 Demographic characteristics of Northwest County adults, 1990 US Census

Characteristic	Percent	Characteristic	Percent
Age		*Education*	
18–24	12.0	<8th grade	14.9
25–34	16.5	9–12 years	13.9
35–44	13.0	High Sch. Grad.	35.5
45–54	12.9	Some College	17.2
55–64	19.4	College Grad.	11.2
65+	26.0	Post Grad. Work	7.2
Race		*Gender*	
White	75.3	Male	48.5
Nonwhite	24.7	Female	51.5
		Income	
<$14,999	44.9	25–34,999	12.5
15–24,999	25.9	35,000+	16.7

6. Which of the following statements *best* describes county residents?
   a. Older, nonwhite females with modest incomes
   b. Younger, white females with modest incomes
   c. Older, white persons, some with high incomes
   d. Older, white males with modest incomes

7. Which of the following statements *best* describes county residents?
   a. Older persons with modest educational attainment
   b. Older persons with high educational attainment
   c. Older females with high educational attainment
   d. Older males with high educational attainment

8. Which of the following statements *best* describes county residents?
   a. Older persons with modest educational attainment and high incomes
   b. Older persons with modest educational attainment and who are largely female
   c. Older persons with modest educational attainment and modest incomes
   d. Older persons with modest educational attainment, modest incomes, and who differ little regarding gender

Case 2: HIV Risk Categories

After being given the table presented below, you have been asked to analyze these data presented:

Table 1 AIDS, United States and Florida, 1991

	United States[a]		Florida[b]	
	# Cases	% Deaths	# Cases	% Deaths
Case Summary				
# Adult Cases	188,348	64	17,779	64
# Peds. Cases[c]	3,253	53	482	55
Total Cases	191,601	64	18,261	64
Adult Exposure Groups		% Cases		% Cases
Homo/Bisexual Males	110,678	59	9,239	52
IV Drug User (IVDU)	41,963	22	3,721	21
Homo/Bisexual IVDU	12,334	7	1,096	6
Hemophiliac	1,597	1	89	1
Heterosexual contact	10,636	6	2,591	15
Transfusion related	4,147	2	488	3
None of the above	6,993	4	555	3
Race/Ethnicity (All)				
White (Non-Hispanic)	103,502	54	8,716	48
Black (Non-Hispanic)	55,181	29	7,064	39
Hispanic	30,964	16	2,446	13
Other	1,486	1	23	0
Sex (Adult Cases)				

	United States[a]		Florida[b]	
	# Cases	**% Deaths**	**# Cases**	**% Deaths**
Male	169,067	90	15,138	85
Female	19,281	10	2,641	15

[a]Cumulative as of 8/31/91; [b]Cumulative as of 9/30/91; [c]<13 years old.
Source: Table 2, The Florida HIV/AIDS Surveillance Report. Disease Control and AIDS Prevention, State Health Office. October, 1991.

9. Which race or ethnic group comprises the largest number of AIDS cases in the United States?
   a. White, Non-Hispanic   c. Hispanic
   b. Black, Non-Hispanic   d. Other

10. What percent of total cases in the US are pediatric in nature?   *ped*
    a. 1.73%   c. 1.70%   *total cases*
    b. 2.71%   d. 0.45%   *1.69 − 1.70*

11. What is the percentage of cases related to IVDU in Florida?
    a. 22%   c. 27%
    b. 21%   d. 29%

DISCUSSION QUESTIONS

1. You have been asked to prepare a public information campaign concerning HIV/AIDS prevention. From the data presented in Case 2, Table 1, describe the target population for your campaign. Also, include a justification as to why you selected particular demographics.

2. Explain the difference between predisposing, enabling, and need variables.

3. When comparing the results of various studies, what might you examine before deciding whether the studies are comparable?

4. Contact a few public and private health related organizations in your town to see what types of demographic information they might have available.

6

Health Planning Methods: Epidemiology

Chapter Objectives:

1. Describe epidemiologic variables commonly used in health planning.
2. Read and interpret epidemiologic data commonly used in health planning.
3. Apply descriptive statistics to demographic and epidemiologic data.
4. Summarize descriptive data into tables, charts, and graphs.

According to Henderson and MacStravic (1982, p. 22) the "analytic and thinking aspects of both planning and administration have three requirements:

a. evaluating existing and predicted problems, threats, and opportunities in the organization and/or its environment, assuming the absence of intervention;
b. identifying, selecting, and using interventions designed to move the organization and the community it serves in some desired direction (or keep it from moving in an undesired one); and
c. monitoring the current state of affairs to check whether interventions were successful and whether additional problems, threats, and opportunities have arisen."

Henderson and MacStravic (1982, p. 23) argue that the "logic of epidemiology is applicable to all three." Hence, epidemiology has been included as a health planning method.

EPIDEMIOLOGY: AN INTRODUCTION

Epidemiologic data can be useful in (a) monitoring the progress of an epidemic, (b) identifying potential service populations and needed services, (c) setting program priorities, (d) determining program size and scope, and (e) evaluating program impact. Demographic variables are very important in the application of epidemiology in health planning.

Sources of epidemiological data include: (a) *The Morbidity and Mortality Weekly Report* (Centers for Disease Control and Prevention, Atlanta), (b) *Monthly Vital Statistics Report* (National Center for Health Statistics, Hyattsville, MD), (c) *Advance Data* (National Center for Health Statistics, Hyattsville, MD), (d) state vital statistics reports (local or state health department), and (e) reports from the local or state health planning agency. Professional and scholarly journals include the *American Journal of Epidemiology*, the *American Journal of Public Welfare*, the *Journal of the American Medical Association [JAMA]*, *Epidemiologic Reviews*, and the *International Journal of Epidemiology*.

Last (1988, p. 42) has defined epidemiology as, "the study of the distribution and determinants of health-related states or events in specified populations, and the application of this study to the control of health problems." Epidemiology concerns itself with measuring disease mortality (death), morbidity (illness), and/or disability within human populations, however defined.

Traditionally, epidemiology has been divided into three subclassifications. Last (1988, pp. 5–6) provides the following definition of analytical epidemiology, "[It is] designed to examine associations, commonly putative or hypothesized causal relationships. [A]n analytic study is usually concerned with identifying or measuring the effects of risk factors, or is concerned with the health effects of specific exposure(s) [and unlike] descriptive [epidemiology], does not test hypotheses." Experimental epidemiology is defined by Last (1988, p. 45) as, "equated with randomized control trials."

Analytic and experimental epidemiology need more discussion and explanation than can be presented here. For more information, see the books *Foundations of Epidemiology* by Lilienfeld and Lilienfeld (1980), *Making Sense of Data: A Self-Instruction Manual on the Interpretation of Epidemiological Data* by Abramson (1988), or *Community Health Analysis* by Dever (1991).

Descriptive epidemiology is defined as, "[the] study of the amount and distribution of disease within a population by person, place, and time" (Mausner and Bahn, 1974, p. 43). While the following list is not all inclusive, the variables of person, time, and place may include:

Person	Time	Place
age	hour	zip code
race	weekday	census tract
gender	month	city
ethnic group	year	state
occupation	decade	clinic

At the operations level, concern is usually with implementing a single project or program. By using descriptive techniques, data can be analyzed and organized in such a way as to present a "snap shot" of the event or circumstance of interest. The resulting information and understanding can guide program design, resource allocation, and program management decisions.

This discussion is confined to descriptive epidemiology: first examining commonly utilized indices (rates, ratios, and proportions) and second, exploring applications of descriptive epidemiology to health planning.

INDICES: RATES

There are principally two types of rates utilized in descriptive epidemiology: (a) incidence rates and (b) prevalence rates which are applied in the context of mortality, morbidity, and disability. Rates may be either crude, cause specific, or case specific. Crude rates are those which reflect morbidity and/or mortality without reference to a specific disease, condition, or set of cases, e.g., crude death rate per 100,000 population. Cause specific rates are those with reference to a specific disease or condition, e.g., AIDS death rate per 100,000 population. Case specific rates are those with reference to a specific epidemiological investigation, e.g., AIDS case fatality rate between 1987 and 1991 in Miami. Frequently used rates, ratios, and proportions are found in Appendix 6.A.

Incidence Rates

Austin and Werner (1974, p. 61) defined incidence as "a measurement of only the new cases of a disease or other event occurring during a given period." New cases of a disease can occur either by onset of the disease among members of the defined population or via immigration of those already ill into the population. The formula which is usually used to compute an incidence rate is:

New period at given [handwritten annotation]

$$\frac{\text{\# of new events in a specified time period}}{\text{\# of persons exposed (or at risk) during the specified period}} \times 10^n$$

Where: 10^n equals the constant which may be expressed as cases per 1,000 or 100,000 population

Pretend that during 1990 there were 11,250 new cases of lung cancer in Florida and we know through the behavioral risk factor surveillance reporting system that there were an estimated 3,400,000 Florida smokers on July 1, 1990. (The behavioral risk factor surveillance reporting system is an on-going state-wide telephone survey which is conducted to examine the health behaviors of US residents, including those who live in Florida.) For illustrative purposes, we have determined that we want to know what is the lung cancer incidence rate among Florida smokers. Let's compute:

# of new events: 11,250 lung cancer cases in 1990
# of persons at risk: 3,400,000 smokers in 1990
specified time period: 1990 (one year)
constant: 100,000 population (i.e., smokers)

$$\frac{11,250}{3,400,000} \times 100,000 = 331$$

Thus, we can see that the 1990 incidence rate for lung cancer among Florida smokers was 331/100,000 population. In other words, in 1990, for every 100,000 Florida smokers 331 developed a new case of lung cancer. This is a cause specific incidence rate, as no formal epidemiological investigation was being conducted.

An attack rate is an incidence rate expressed as a percent. It is applied to a specific population for a limited period of time. Using data from our example, we compute the lung cancer attack rate to be .33% (11,250 divided by 3,400,000).

Prevalence Rates

Austin and Werner (1974, p. 62) defined prevalence rate as, "a measurement of all cases of disease or other events prevailing at a given time. It includes new cases and old cases." According to Ferrara, (1980, p. 137) there are two types of prevalence rates. Point prevalance rates measure prevalence at a given instant in time, e.g., a single day, while period prevalence rates consider a specified period of time, e.g., an entire month.

The formula for computing a prevalance rate is:

$$\frac{\text{\# of new + old cases during a specified time period}}{\text{population at risk during the specified time period}} \times 10^n$$

New and old given period

For example, return to the lung cancer pretend data:

# of new events: 11,250 lung cancer cases in 1990
# of old events: 20,000 lung cancer cases in 1990
persons at risk: 3,400,000 smokers in 1990
specified time period: 1990 (one year)
constant: 100,000 population (i.e., smokers)

$$\frac{31,250}{3,400,000} \times 100,000 = 919/100,000$$

The lung cancer prevalence rate in 1990 was 919 cases for every 100,000 Florida smokers. This is a cause specific period prevalence rate.

Comparing Rates

While singular incidence and prevalence rates provide us with useful data, they are more useful when compared to similar rates for compatible populations or samples. For example, we know the 1985 Florida lung cancer morbidity incidence (pretend data) [1985 = 287 cases/100,000] and prevalence [1985 = 801 cases/100,000] rates.

By comparing 1985 and 1990 rates, we can see that lung cancer morbidity has increased among Florida smokers as well as lung cancer mortality. Thus, the more data we have, the more detailed and precise can be our epidemiological descriptions of a health problem, target population, or some other situation of interest.

INDICES: RATIOS

Austin and Werner (1974, p. 62) defined ratio as "used to express the relationship of one number to another."

In our example, we find that new male lung cancer cases in 1990 were 8,231 and new female lung cancer cases were 3,019. To compute the ratio of new male to female lung cancer cases, we divide 3,019 into 8,231, which equals 2.73. Thus, the ratio of new male to female lung cancer cases in 1990 was 2.73:1. By convention, "1" is always to the right of ":" and the value to the left of the ":" is rounded to two decimal places.

INDICES: PROPORTIONS

While it is often very beneficial to convert data to rates, ratios, and measures of central tendency so as to be able to compare samples drawn from compatible populations, compare groups over time, or trace changes in health seeking behaviors between and among groups, proportional data are instructive. A proportion is a percentage.

By way of illustration, return to our example in the ratio discussion. There were 11,250 new cases of lung cancer in 1990. Seventy-three percent (8,231) were male and 27% (3,019) were female. By convention, sentences do not start with a percentage expressed as a number, e.g., 73%.

INDICES: MEASURES OF CENTRAL TENDENCY

There are three measures of central tendency used in descriptive epidemiology. These are: (a) mean, (b) median, and (c) mode. An explanation of each follows:

Mean

The mean is just another way of saying average and is symbolized by $\overline{X}$. To compute a mean, all we do is add up all the numbers of interest and then divide by the number of numbers we add up. For example, suppose we determined that the following lung cancer mortality was observed during the past five years:

Year	# Deaths	Year	# Deaths
1985:	8,972	1988:	13,987
1986:	9,732	1989:	13,567
1987:	10,324		56,582

We want to know the average number of deaths due to lung cancer over the past five years. So, we divide 56,582 by 5 which equals 11,316.40. In 1990, 12,350 lung cancer deaths were recorded. These are artificial data.

Median

The median is the category or actual score above which 50% of the cases fall and below which 50% of the cases fall. For example, consider these artificial 1990 lung cancer morbidity data:

Age	# Cases	Age	# Cases
1–18	0	50–54	1,989
19–24	1	55–59	2,001
25–29	65	60–64	2,321 –
30–34	187	65–69	1,000
35–40	987	70+	191
41–44	1,019		
45–49	1,489		

First, we divide 11,250 by 2 so that we determine what is 50 percent of the numbers. We compute the quotient to be 5,625. Next, we count up from the bottom until we locate the age cohort where the 5,625th case occurred, which is 50–54. Next, we compute the mid-point of the 50–54 age cohort which is 52.5 years. Thus, we know that approximately 50 percent of male lung cancer morbidity occurred before and after 52.5 years.

Of couse, this method does not produce an exact median; to do that we would have to list all 11,250 cases with the corresponding age to get an exact median. The 1990 female lung cancer case median age was 62.5 years (computations not shown). For males, it was 52.5 years.

Mode

The mode is the number or category wherein the number which occurs most often is found. From our median example, we find the mode to be the 60–64 age cohort, as it contains 2,321 cases. With respect to male lung cancer morbidity in 1990, the modal cohort was 60–64 years. The 1990 female lung cancer morbidity modal cohort was 60–64 years (computations not shown). It is not uncommon for the mean, median, and mode to vary. *age group with greatest statistic*

PULLING IT ALL TOGETHER _____

A number of descriptive epidemiological indices have been computed or given. These are summarized below:

    1990 Incidence Rate: 331 cases/100,000 population
    1990 Prevalence Rate: 919 cases/100,000 population
    1990 Male/Female Case Morbidity Ratio: 2.73:1 *onset*
    1990 Male & Female Morbidity Proportions: 73% male
                                              27% female
    1985–89 Mean Lung Cancer Mortality: 11,316.40
    1990 Lung Cancer Mortality: 12,350 *death*
    1990 Male Lung Cancer Case Median Age: 52.5 years
    1990 Male Lung Cancer Case Modal Cohort: 60–64 years
    1990 Female Lung Cancer Case Median Age: 62.5 years
    1990 Female Lung Cancer Case Modal Cohort: 60–64 years

We are now able to describe lung cancer morbidity and mortality among Florida smokers in epidemiological terms using the demographic variable, gender. Based on the above data, we can see that more males developed cases of lung cancer than females and at an earlier age. Lung cancer mortality in 1990 (12,350 deaths) was greater than the five-year (85–89) average of 11,316.40 deaths.

A possible use for such data in planning a prevention program would be to target males before age 53 and females before age 62 with smoking cessation messages which appeal to those age groups. More messages should be targeted to males than females given the greater male lung cancer morbidity experience. Given the documented growth of lung cancer morbidity and mortality, planners should propose that acute care capacity be expanded, if necessary.

There has emerged a specialization, behavioral epidemiology, within the science of epidemiology. Behavioral epidemiologists study the impact of behavior on disease incidence or prevalence and/or on health status. By understanding the relationship between various behaviors and health status, appropriate interventions can be planned, implemented, and evaluated. This is very important given the relationship among health related behaviors, health status, and health costs.

In 1981, The Centers for Disease Control and Prevention (CDC) initiated the Behavioral Risk Factor Surveillance System (BRFSS). The purpose of the BRFSS is to describe American adult health behaviors and the relationship of those behaviors to health status (Remington, Smith, Williamson, Anda, Gentry, and Hogelin, 1988). BRFSS data are routinely reported in the *Morbidity and Mortality Weekly Report*. Many participating states issue reports as well.

PRESENTING DESCRIPTIVE EPIDEMIOLOGICAL DATA

There are several suggested methods for presenting descriptive epidemiological data. These are: (a) tables, (b) graphs, and (c) charts. These presentation guidelines apply to the presentation of demographic and health services research data as well. Following is a discussion of each method, including commonly accepted guidelines.

Presenting Data: Tables

Ferrara (1980, p. 89) has provided guidance in constructing tables for the presentation of data. These guidelines are quoted:

a. Tables should be as simple as possible. Two or three small tables are preferable to a single large table containing many details or variables. Generally, three variables are the maximum number which can be read with ease.
b. Tables should be self-explanatory. Codes, abbreviations, or symbols should be explained in detail in a footnote. Each row and each column should be labeled concisely and clearly. The specific units of measure for data should be given. The title should be clear, concise, and to the point. Answers: what? when? where? Totals should be shown (if applicable).

c. The title is commonly separated from the body of the table by lines or spaces. In small tables, vertical lines separating the columns may not be necessary.

d. If data are not original, their source should be given in a footnote.

Table 6.1 is a reproduction of a data table from the previously mentioned Collier County, Florida study. Its purpose is to illustrate an application of Ferrara's guidelines in presenting epidemiological data.

An estimated 13,764 adult (18+ years), permanent Collier County, Florida residents (21% of the adult population), had been diagnosed as being hypertensive. Married (24.6% at risk) females (23.5%) were at greater risk for being hypertensive than unmarried (12.4%) males (18.2%). Those with less than nine years of education were

Table 6.1[a] Characteristics of current hypertensives
Collier County, Florida, 1985

Characteristic	% at Risk[b]	Characteristic	% at Risk
Race		Education	
White	21.3	<9 years	40.5
Black	23.4	10–12 years	18.8
Hispanic	14.9	High Sch. Grad.	16.8
		Tech. School	13.7
Marital Status		Some College	22.0
Married	24.6	College Grad.	27.3
Unmarried	12.4	Post Grad.	14.2
Gender		Income	
Male	18.2	<$10,000	25.3
Female	23.5	10–15,000	16.2
		15–20,000	20.0
Age		20–25,000	18.3
18–24	3.8	25–35,000	18.5
25–34	6.4	>35,000	23.9
35–44	17.3		
45–54	17.9		
55–64	30.8		
65+	35.9		

[a]Data columns will not total to 100 percent.
[b]The "% at risk" label means that a respondent reported being told more than once that he or she had elevated blood pressure. For example, while 23.5% of females were at risk for hypertension, 76.5% were not.
Source: Hale, C. D. (1986). *1985 Behavioral Health Risks of Collier County, Florida Adults.* Naples: Collier County Public Health Department.

most at risk for being hypertensive, while those with the most education were at the least risk. Of course, the risk for hypertension increases with age, but the effect of income on risk status is uncertain as the data are too mixed to provide any useful information.

Presenting Data: Graphs

Ferrara (1980, p. 92) has defined graphing as, "a method of showing quantitative data using a coordinate system (for our purposes, usually x and y)." He has advanced the following as general graphing principles:

a. The simplest graphs are the most effective. No more lines or symbols should be used in a single graph than the eye can easily follow. Every graph should be self-explanatory.
b. The title may be placed either at the top or bottom of the graph.
c. When more than one variable is shown on a graph, each should be clearly differentiated by means of legends or keys.
d. No more coordinate lines should be used than are necessary to guide the eye.
e. Lines of the graph itself should be heavier than other coordinate lines.
f. Frequency is usually represented on the vertical scale and method of classification on the horizontal scale.
g. On an arithmetic scale, equal increments on the scale must represent equal numerical units.
h. Scale divisions should be clearly indicated as well as the units into which the scale is divided.

From the several graphing options presented by Ferrara (1980, pp. 92–102), three are particularly useful. The arithmetic scale line graph is "one where an equal distance represents an equal quantity anywhere on the [y] axis, but not . . . between the axes [x and y] (p. 94)." See Figure 6.1.

Ferrara (1980, p. 96) described the histogram (Figure 6.2) as, "a graph used only for presenting frequency distribution of quantitative data. There is no space between the cells . . . on a histogram." It is customary to include only one set of data in a histogram.

Do not confuse a histogram with a bar chart which has space between the cells.

A frequency polygon (Figure 6.3) is used to present at least one set of data. It is common to use two or more sets of data. Constructed from a histogram, the midpoints of a class interval (how data are grouped) may be connected by a straight line. It is best to use class intervals of equal sizes. These are useful in showing relationships.

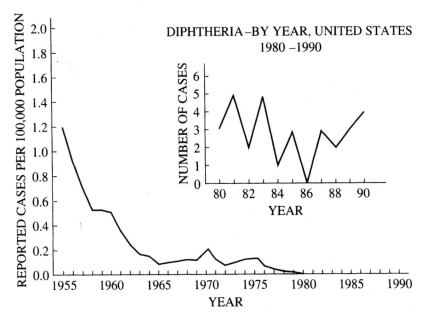

Figure 6.1 Diptheria by year, United States, 1955–1990
Source: Summary of Notifiable Diseases, United States, 1990, p. 22. Centers for Disease Control, 1991.

Presenting Data: Charts

Ferrara (1980, p. 102) has defined a chart as "a method of presenting statistical information symbolically using only one coordinate." The most commonly employed chart is the bar chart (Figure 6.4). Ferrara (p. 103) suggested the following construction guidelines:

a. The bar chart has cells, all the same column width.
b. There are also spaces between the columns.
c. The bars can be arranged either vertically or horizontally.
d. It is best to arrange the bars in either descending or ascending order for ease of reading.
e. Never use a scale break.
f. Columns may be shaded, hatched, or colored to emphasize differences between the bars.
g. The bars should be labeled at the bottom of the chart and not in the middle.
h. Group related information together but be sure to space between groups.

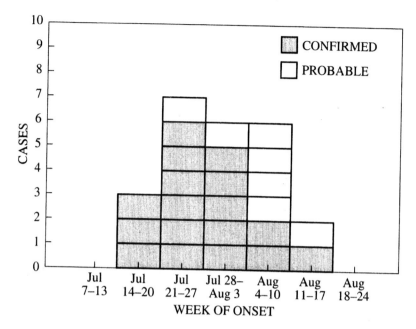

Figure 6.2 Cases of St. Louis encephalitis by week of onset, Pine Bluff, AK, July and August, 1991
Source: Morbidity and Mortality Weekly Report, *40*, (35), p. 606. Centers for Disease Control, 1991.

The chief advantage of the bar chart is its simplicity.

Another commonly utilized chart is the pie chart (Figure 6.5), which is useful in displaying proportions. Ferrara (1980, p. 107) has suggested the following guidelines in preparing a pie chart:

a. Start at the 12 o'clock position and arrange segments in the order of their magnitude, starting with the largest value.
b. Proceed clockwise around the chart.
c. To convert from a percentage to degrees, multiply the percentage by 3.6.

It should be noted that many computer programs will generate charts and graphs automatically. It may be useful to purchase one of these graphics programs in order to avoid constructing a chart or graph by hand which can be a time consuming (and frustrating) process.

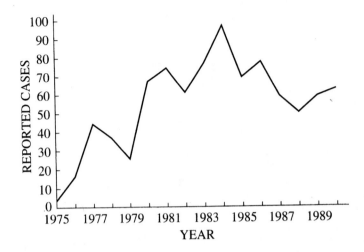

Figure 6.3 Infant botulism by year, United States, 1975–1990.
Source: Summary of Notifiable Diseases, United States, 1990, p. 21. Centers for Disease Control, 1991.

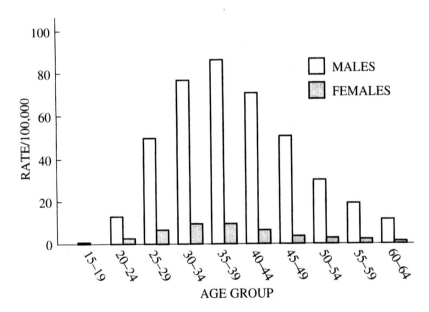

Figure 6.4 Acquired immunodeficiency syndrome (AIDS) annual rates per 100,000 population by selected age group and sex for reported cases, United States, 1990.
Source: Summary of Notifiable Diseases, United States, 1990, p. 16. Centers for Disease Control, 1991.

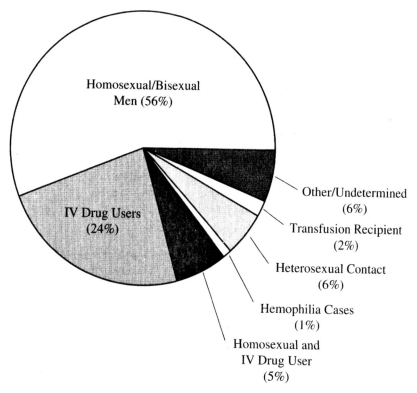

Figure 6.5 Acquired immunodeficiency syndrome (AIDS) reported adult/ adolescent cases, by exposure category, United States, 1990.
Source: Summary of Notifiable Diseases, United States, 1990, p. 16. Centers for Disease Control, 1991.

SUMMARY

The application of epidemiology to describe the health status of a community or group provides planners and managers with valuable information for decision making. Descriptive epidemiology is used to describe health status according to the variables of time, person, and place. The various indices employed include measures of central tendency (mean, median, and mode), incidence rates, prevalence rates, ratios, and proportions.

Epidemiological data may be summarized and presented in tables, histograms, frequency polygons, bar charts, and pie charts. There are guidelines for the construction of tables, graphs, and charts which should be followed. These presentation devices are powerful. When constructing a table, graph, or chart, keep the image as simple and as tidy as possible.

Appendix 6.A

Frequently used rates, ratios, and proportions

No.	Description of Measure	Numerator (x)	Denominator (y)	Expressed Per Number At Risk (k)
	NATALITY			
1.	*Birth Rate* Crude; specific for age of mother, sex of child, socioeconomic status, etc.	Number of live births reported during a given time interval	Estimated mid-interval population	1,000
2.	*Fertility Rate* (a) *Theoretical Purposes*	Number of live births reported during a given time interval from mothers aged 15–44 years	Estimated number of women in age group 15–44 years at mid-interval	1,000
	(b) *Current Usage* Crude; specific for age of mother, race, socioeconomic status, etc.	Number of live births reported during a given time interval	Estimated number of women in age group 15–44 years at mid-interval	1,000
3.	*Low Birth Weight Ratio* Crude; specific for age of mother, race, socioeconomic area, etc.	Number of live births under 2,500 grams (or 5½ lbs.) during a given time interval	Number of live births reported during the same time interval	100
	MORBIDITY			
4.	*Incidence Rate* Crude by cause; specific for age, race, sex, socioeconomic area, stage of disease, etc.	Number of new cases of a specified disease reported during a given time interval	Estimated mid-interval population	Variable: 10^x where $x = 2, 3, 4, 5, 6$
5.	*Attack Rate* Crude by cause; specific for age, race, sex, socioeconomic area, etc.	Number of new cases of a specified disease reported during a specific time interval	Total population at risk during the same time interval	Variable: 10^x where $x = 2, 3, 4, 5, 6$

No.	Description of Measure	Numerator (x)	Denominator (y)	Expressed Per Number At Risk (k)
6.	*Point Prevalence Rate (Ratio)* Crude by cause; specific for age, race, sex, socio-economic area, stage of disease, etc.	Number of current cases, new and old, of a specified disease existing at a given point in time	Estimated population at the same point in time	Variable: 10^x where $x = 2, 3, 4, 5, 6$
7.	*Period (Case-Load) Prevalence Rate (Ratio)* Crude by cause; specific for age, race, sex, socio-economic area, stage of disease, etc.	Number of current cases, new and old, of a specified disease occurring during a given time interval	Estimated mid-interval population	Variable: 10^x where $x = 2, 3, 4, 5, 6$
	MORTALITY			
8.	*Crude Death Rate* Crude; specific for age, race, sex, socio-economic area, etc.	Total number of deaths reported during a given time interval	Estimated mid-interval population	1,000
9.	*Cause-Specific Death Rate* or *Cause of Death Rate* Crude by cause; specific for age, race, sex, socio-economic area, etc.	Number of deaths assigned to a specific cause during a given time interval	Estimated mid-interval population	100,000
10.	*Cause-Specific Death Ratio* or *Cause of Death Ratio* or *Proportional Mortality Ratio* Crude by cause; specific for age, race, sex, socio-economic area, etc.	Number of deaths assigned to a specified cause during a given time interval	Total number of deaths from all causes reported during the same interval	100 or 1,000

No.	Description of Measure	Numerator (x)	Denominator (y)	Expressed Per Number At Risk (k)
11.	*Case Fatality Rate (Ratio) Death-to-Case Ratio* Crude; specific for age, race, sex, socioeconomic area, etc.	Number of deaths assigned to a specified disease during a given time interval	Number of new cases of that disease reported during the same time interval	100
12.	(a) *Fetal Death Rate I* Crude; specific for age of mother, race, socioeconomic area, etc.	Number of fetal deaths of 28 weeks or more gestation reported during a given time interval	Number of fetal deaths of 28 weeks or more gestation reported during the same time interval plus the number of live births occurring during the same time interval	1,000
	(b) *Fetal Death Rate II* Crude; specific for age of mother, race, socioeconomic area, etc.	Number of fetal deaths of 20 weeks or more gestation reported during a given time interval	Number of fetal deaths of 20 weeks or more gestation reported during the same time interval plus the number of live births occurring during the same time interval	1,000
13.	(a) *Fetal Death Ratio I* Crude; specific for age of mother, race, socioeconomic area, etc.	Number of fetal deaths of 28 weeks or more gestation reported during a given time interval	Number of live births reported during the same time interval	1,000
	(b) *Fetal Death Ratio II*			

No.	Description of Measure	Numerator (x)	Denominator (y)	Expressed Per Number At Risk (k)
	Crude; specific for age of mother, race, socioeconomic area, etc.	Number of fetal deaths of 20 weeks or more gestation reported during a given time interval	Number of live births reported during the same time interval	1,000
14.	(a) *Perinatal Mortality Rate I*			
	Crude; specific for age of mother, race, socioeconomic area, etc.	Number of fetal deaths of 28 weeks or more gestation reported during a given time interval plus the reported number of infant deaths under seven days of life during the same time interval	Number of fetal deaths of 28 weeks or more gestation reported during the same time interval. plus the number of live births occurring during the same time interval	1,000
	(b) *Perinatal Mortality Rate II*			
	Crude; specific for age of mother, sex, socioeconomic area, etc.	Number of fetal deaths of 20 weeks or more gestation reported during a given time interval plus the reported number of infant deaths under 28 days of life during the same time interval	Number of fetal deaths of 20 weeks or more gestation reported during the same time interval plus the number of live births reported during the same time interval	1,000
15.	*Infant Mortality Rate*			
	Crude; specific for race, sex, socio-economic area; birth weight, cause of death, etc.	Number of deaths under 1 year of age reported during a given time interval	Number of live births reported during the same time interval	1,000
16.	*Neonatal Mortality Rate*			
	Crude; specific for race, sex, socioeconomic area, birth weight, cause of death, etc.	Number of deaths under 28 days of age reported during a given time interval	Number of live births reported during the same time interval	1,000

No.	Description of Measure	Numerator (x)	Denominator (y)	Expressed Per Number At Risk (k)
17.	*Postneonatal Mortality Rate*			
	(a) *Theoretical Purposes*	Number of deaths from 28 days of age up to, but not including, 1 year of age, reported during a given time interval	Number of live births reported during the same time interval less the number of deaths under 28 days of age	1,000
	(b) *Current Usage* Crude; specific for race, sex, socio-economic area, cause of death, etc.	Number of deaths from 28 days of age up to, but not including, 1 year of age, reported during a given time interval	Number of live births reported during the same time interval	1,000
18.	*Maternal Mortality Rate* Crude; specific for age of mother, race, socioeconomic area, etc.	Number of deaths assigned to causes related to pregnancy during a given time interval	Number of live births reported during the same time interval	10,000

REVIEW AND APPLICATION QUESTIONS

Directions. Read each question very carefully before selecting your answer. There is one correct answer for each question.

1. The definition, "the study of the distribution and determinants of health-related states or events in specified populations, and the application of this study to control of health problems," refers to:
   a. Demography   c. Evaluation
   b. Financial   d. Epidemiology

2. The branch of epidemiology, whose major characteristics include person, time, and place, is:
   a. Analytical epidemiology
   b. Experimental epidemiology

c. Descriptive epidemiology
d. Quasi-experimental epidemiology

3. The branch of epidemiology which is designed to examine associations and is " . . . concerned with identifying or measuring the effects of risk factors" is:
   a. Experimental epidemiology
   b. Descriptive epidemiology
   c. Quasi-experimental epidemiology
   d. Analytical epidemiology

4. The branch of epidemiology which is equated with randomized control trials and classical laboratory research is:
   a. Descriptive epidemiology
   b. Quasi-experimental epidemiology
   c. Analytical epidemiology
   d. Experimental epidemiology

5. When reviewing and considering the use of any type of data (demographic or epidemiologic), one can assess data through all of the following means EXCEPT:
   a. Compare suspect data to what was expected
   b. Compare suspect data to existing data whose quality is unknown
   c. Evaluate suspect data for compatibility with what is already known
   d. Examine suspect data for consistency within itself

6. The epidemiologic indice which is defined as "the number of new cases within a specified population in a given time period" is:
   a. Prevalence rate   c. Proportion
   b. Incidence rate   d. Ratio

7. The epidemiologic indice which is defined as "the total number of persons who have an attribute or disease at any given time period" is:
   a. Incidence rate   c. Ratio
   b. Proportion   d. Prevalence rate

8. The epidemiologic indice which is defined as "an expression of the relationship between a numerator and denominator where the two are usually separate and distinct quantities, neither being included in the other" is:
   a. Proportion   c. Prevalence rate
   b. Ratio   d. Incidence rate

9. Each of the following are measures of central tendency EXCEPT:
   a. Mean   c. Standard deviation
   b. Mode   d. Median

Case 1: Diabetes in XYZ County

Read the following epidemiologic report concerning diabetes in XYZ County and answer the following questions.

West XYZ County

1990 Incidence Rate: 57/100,000 pop.
1990 Prevalence Rate: 153/100,000 pop.
1990 Male/Female Mortality Ratio: 2:1
1990 Male Diabetes Onset Mean Age: 57
1990 Male Diabetes Mortality Median Cohort: 60–64 —
1990 Female Diabetes Onset Mean Age: 63
1990 Female Diabetes Mortality Median Cohort: 60–64

East XYZ County

1990 Incidence Rate: 33/100,000 pop.
1990 Prevalence Rate: 217/100,000 pop.
1990 Male/Female Mortality Ratio: 3:1 .
1990 Male Diabetes Onset Mean Age: 57
1990 Male Diabetes Mortality Median Cohort: 55–59
1990 Female Diabetes Onset Mean Age: 67
1990 Female Diabetes Mortality Median Cohort: 60–64 -

10. Which side of XYZ County seems to have the most cases of diabetes?
    a. West
    b. East
    c. Both appear to be about equal
    d. Insufficient information provided

11. Which side of XYZ County seems to have the most new cases of diabetes?
    a. West
    b. East
    c. Both appear to be about equal
    d. Insufficient information provided

12. In which side of the county do males seem to die earlier from diabetes?
    a. West
    b. East
    c. Both appear to be about equal
    d. Insufficient information provided

13. In which side of the county do females seem to die earlier from diabetes?
    a. West
    b. East
    c. Both appear to be about equal
    d. Insufficient information provided

14. Which side of the county seems to experience the greatest difference in gender related death?
    a. West
    b. East
    c. Both appear to be about equal
    d. Insufficient information provided

Case 2: Heart Disease in XYZ County

Read the following epidemiologic report concerning heart disease in XYZ County and answer the following questions.

West XYZ County

1990 Incidence Rate: 167/100,000 pop.
1990 Prevalence Rate: 317/100,000 pop.
1990 Male/Female Mortality Ratio: 2:1
1990 Male Heart Disease Onset Mean Age: 67
1990 Male Heart Disease Mortality Median Cohort: 65–69
1990 Female Heart Disease Onset Mean Age: 71
1990 Female Heart Disease Mortality Median Cohort: 70–74

East XYZ County

1990 Incidence Rate: 173/100,000 pop.
1990 Prevalence Rate: 315/100,000 pop.
1990 Male/Female Mortality Ratio: 1:1
1990 Male Heart Disease Onset Mean Age: 65
1990 Male Heart Disease Mortality Median Cohort: 60–64
1990 Female Heart Disease Onset Mean Age: 67
1990 Female Heart Disease Mortality Median Cohort: 70–74

15. Given those data presented above, which side of XYZ County seems to have the most cases of newly diagnosed cases of heart disease?
    a. West
    b. East
    c. Both appear to be about equal
    d. Insufficient information provided

16. Given those data presented above, which side of XYZ County seems to be least affected by heart disease morbidity?
    a. West
    b. East
    c. Both appear to be about equal
    d. Insufficient information provided

17. Given those data presented above, in which side of the county do females seem to be the most affected by heart disease morbidity?
    a. West
    b. East
    c. Both appear to be about equal
    d. Insufficient information provided

18. Given those data presented above, in which side of the county do males seem to be most affected by heart disease mortality?
    a. West
    (b.) East
    c. Both appear to be about equal
    d. Insufficient information provided

19. Given those data presented above, which side of the county seems to experience the greatest difference in gender related onset?
    (a.) West
    b. East
    c. Both appear to be about equal
    d. Insufficient information provided

DISCUSSION QUESTIONS

1. Pick a disease or health problem in which you have an interest or select one from Appendix 2.A. Research its incidence and/or prevalence in your community. Describe the disease or health problem according to person, time and place.

2. Summarize your data from question one into tables, graphs, and/or charts. Once this has been done, prepare a brief report for presentation and discussion.

3. Research computer software programs that can generate graphics. Prepare a list which includes name, price, vendor, computer system requirements, and capabilities. Which one would you select and why?

7

Health Planning Methods: Health Services Research

Chapter Objectives:

1. Describe health sevice research variables commonly used in health planning.
2. Read and interpret descriptive health services research data commonly reported in health planning.
3. Describe the survey research process.
4. Describe a recommended format for a research report.

Often, at the operational level within healthcare organizations, planners are faced with issues which involve increasing market share, implementing a new technology, starting a new program, or turning around a declining patient census. Health services research can assist the planner in (a) describing the current state of affairs, (b) selecting interventions or strategies to attain desired goals and objectives, (c) monitoring plan implementation and/or program performance, (d) assessing quality of care or other quality interests, and (e) knowing when desired conditions are present or when goals and objectives have been attained. The use of health services research (HSR) methods can improve and strengthen the operational health planning process by providing detailed, accurate descriptions of health services organization, distribution, delivery, and utilization. Accordingly, the purpose of the following discussion is to acquaint you with descriptive applications of health services research so as to enable you to evaluate the quality of HSR generated data. Also, you will be better equipped to conduct similar assessments of descriptive demographic and epidemiological studies and data.

Presented in this chapter is a discussion of (a) descriptive health services research, (b) descriptive HSR indices and applications, (c) the survey research process, and (d) HSR design considerations.

DESCRIPTIVE HEALTH SERVICES RESEARCH _____

Introduction

HSR may be defined as the application of research principles and methods to the study of health services organization, distribution, delivery, utilization, management, and finance. Data collection methods include surveys, interviews, and document reviews. HSR data analysis techniques include application of descriptive and/or inferential statistics. While not included within this discussion, HSR also includes quasi-experimental and experimental designs. If you are interested in such designs you may find *Methodological Advances in Health Services Research* by DeFriese, Ricketts, and Stein (1989) and *Experimental and Quasi-Experimental Designs for Research* by Campbell and Stanley (1963) to be instructive.

For an illustration of descriptive data which may be produced through HSR methods, refer to Table 7.1. Nelson, (1991, p. 1) reported that adolescent females visited physicians' offices more than adolescent males, while African-Americans (i.e., Blacks) made more visits than other non-white races in 1985. Office visits, as a function of age, appeared to be variable. Knowing who obtains health care, how much of it is obtained,

Table 7.1 Office visits by sex, race, and ethnicity
United States, 1985

Variables	All Ages	11–20 Years	11–14 Years	15–20 Years
Number in 1000s	636,386	58,996	19,360	39,637
		Percent Distribution		
All Visits	100.00	100.00	100.00	100.00
Sex				
Female	60.89	57.39	50.07	60.96
Male	39.11	42.61	49.93	39.04
Race				
White	89.96	89.29	90.78	88.57
Black	8.19	8.76	7.47	9.39
Other	1.84	1.95	1.74	2.05
Ethnicity				
Hispanic	6.38	7.52	6.22	8.15
Non-Hispanic	93.62	92.48	93.78	91.85

Source: Nelson, C. *Office Visits by Adolescents*. (Advance Data no 196.) Hyattsville, MD: National Center for Health Statistics, 1991.

and who does not have access provides valuable information in developing health care delivery plans. Having such information enables a health planner to be more precise and efficient.

In order for health service research data to be helpful in program planning and evaluation, it must be relevant, timely, practical, verifiable, easily understood, presented concisely, and presented without bias. The HSR methods, employed, should be applicable to operational problems (or situations); designed to produce data needed to identify problems and generate solutions; as simple as possible; and appropriate for the user's budget, management capacity, and level of technical competence.

HSR Data Sources

Data, generated by health services research, may come from the same sources as demographic and epidemiologic data. Additionally, local health planning agencies, chambers of commerce, state health planning agencies, local health service organizations (public and private), foundations, and other governmental agencies generally have appropriate data.

Other sources of HSR data include scientific and professional journals, trade publications, unpublished studies, and personal files. Particular journal titles include: (a) *Hospital and Health Services Administration*, (b) *International Journal of Health Services*, (c) *Journal of Health Care for the Poor and Underserved*, (d) *HSR* [Health Services Research] and (e) the *American Journal of Public Health*. When collecting data, it may be helpful to make friends and colleagues aware of your search as they may want to provide their assistance.

DESCRIPTIVE HSR INDICES AND APPLICATIONS _____

Aday and Shortell (1988, p. 52) write that there are "four principal dimensions" of health services utilization [research]: type, purpose, time interval, and site. Type refers to the "category of service rendered" (e.g., physician, hospital inpatient, long-term care admission, prescription, or medical equipment use). Purpose "refers to the reason care was sought" (e.g., acute illness, trauma, restorative care, or primary prevention). Time interval refers to contact (e.g., number of persons seeing a dentist in the last year), volume (e.g., total number of services during a time period), and episodic patterns (e.g., care provided in relation to an illness or physician specialty). Site refers to the location of care delivery (physician's office, hospital, or clinic). Utilization data reported, within one or more of these dimensions, is useful in planning and evaluation.

Common indicators or measures associated with health services research include: (a) length of stay (or program participation); (b) service utilization rates (i.e., persons attending or number and types of services provided); (c) percent occupancy (as in a hospital or nursing home); (d) service admission rates (i.e., hospital admissions which could be sorted by disease, condition, or insurance type); and (e) cost data (i.e., budgeting, cost per unit of service, or cost/benefit). Any of these indices can, and often are, sorted by various demographic variables (e.g., age or gender). DeLozier and Gagnon (1991, p. 3) reported there were 692.7 million visits to non-federally employed physicians in 1989. Persons aged 25–44 years made more physician visits in absolute terms than any other age group. Females made more office visits than males, especially those aged 25–44 years old. Generally, the rate of visits per person, per year increased with age. The per person, per visit rate was similar for males and females during the earlier and later years of life. Please refer to Table 7.2.

Such information is useful in drawing a profile of who utilizes services at the organizational level. Such profiles can be used to guide or evaluate marketing efforts through pre- and post-profile comparison. Further, such information can guide resource allocation decisions. For example, a primary care center for women's health is more likely to have higher patient utilization than one for men.

DeLozier and Gagnon (1991, p. 7) provide information concerning office visit duration (Table 7.3). Knowledge of a visit's duration is essential in forecasting service capacity which may have a direct bearing on potential organizational income. If the unit of remuneration is a patient encounter (such as a physician office visit), then the more patient encounters, the higher potential organizational income. It stands to reason that the shorter the visit, the greater the number of daily encounters. To increase organizational service capacity, more physicians could be added or duration of visit could be reduced, thereby allowing for more billable patient encounters per day.

To further describe physician office visits, we again turn to DeLozier and Gagnon (1991, p. 7) who described office visit disposition (Table 7.4). Sixty-one percent of patients were scheduled to return to the physician's office at another specified time, usually requiring the payment of another office visit fee. From an insurance company's perspective, such information can be useful in designing cost-containment strategies, such as capping the amount of reimbursement a physician may receive per procedure or raising the co-payment a patient must pay for each visit to a physician's office (this tends to reduce service utilization). On the organizational level, such information could serve as a basis for budget building.

In Tables 7.2 to 7.4, various aspects of 1989 physician office visits were described. Had additional information been presented, a more complete description would have emerged. With such descriptive information, planning and management decisions can be made with higher degrees of precision, accuracy, and certainty.

THE SURVEY RESEARCH PROCESS

Given the typically immediate need for descriptive data in operations planning and management, the following discussion is delimited to survey research which has the ability to produce data relatively quickly and inexpensively. Rubinson and Neutens

Table 7.2 Number, percent, and annual rate of office visits by patient sex and age
United States, 1989[a]

Sex and Age	# Visits in 1000's	Percent	# per person per year
Both Sexes			
All ages	692,702	100.0	2.8
<15 years	137,502	19.9	2.6
15–24 years	66,868	9.7	1.9
25–44 years	192,593	27.8	2.4
45–64 years	145,160	21.0	3.1
65–74 years	83,692	12.1	4.7
75 years & over	66,888	9.7	5.9
Female			
All ages	417,496	60.3	3.3
<15 years	65,138	9.4	2.5
15–24 years	43,065	6.2	2.4
25–44 years	130,222	18.8	3.2
45–64 years	87,076	12.6	3.6
65–74 years	49,560	7.2	5.0
75 years & over	42,435	6.1	5.9
Male			
All ages	275,206	39.7	2.3
<15 years	72,364	10.4	2.6
15–24 years	23,803	3.4	1.4
25–44 years	62,370	9.0	1.6
45–64 years	58,084	8.4	2.6
65–74 years	34,133	4.9	4.3
75 years & over	24,453	3.5	5.8

[a]Rates are based on estimates of the civilian noninstitutionalized population of the United States on July 1, 1989.
Source: DeLozier, J. E. & Gagnon, R. O. *National Ambulatory Medical Care Survey: 1989 Summary.* (Advance Data no 203.) Hyattsville, MD: National Center for Health Statistics, 1991.

(1987, pp. 96–98) have conveniently summarized the survey research process (presented in adapted form) as follows:

a. *Commencing the survey:* The purpose of the survey is defined and the scope of the survey is determined given the budget, resources, and capacity of the organization planning the survey. These decisions should be reduced to writing and in detail.

Table 7.3 Number and percent of office visits' duration
United States, 1989

Duration	# Visits in 1000's	Percent
All Durations	692,702	100.00
0 minutes[a]	15,484	2.2
1–5 minutes	65,153	9.4
6–10 minutes	191,103	27.6
11–15 minutes	215,017	31.0
16–30 minutes	164,845	23.8
31 or more minutes	41,100	5.9

[a]Represents office visits in which there was no face-to-face contact between patient and the physician.
Source: DeLozier, J. E. & Gagnon, R. O. *National Ambulatory Medical Care Survey: 1989 Summary.*
(Advance Data no 203.) Hyattsville, MD: National Center for Health Statistics, 1991.

b. *Survey design*: At this stage, the sample, data collection device, work flow, data analysis plan, and reporting requirements are specified and recorded in detail.

c. *Construct the data collection device*: Within this stage, the data collection form is constructed. Careful attention should be paid to question or statement form, content, ordering, and presentation.

d. *Pretest the collection device*: Here, the device is pretested with a small group of subjects similar to those in the sample. Pretest subjects should not be included in the subsequent sample. Provide space on the survey form for subjects to offer comments, suggestions, and criticism. Instruct subjects to write comments after completing the survey form. For data collection devices, such as data sheets used in chart audits, instruct coders to make written comments.

Table 7.4 Number and percent of office visit disposition
United States, 1989

Disposition	# Visits in 1000's	Percent
No followup planned	66,377	9.6
Return at specified time	424,583	61.3
Return if needed	160,282	23.1
Telephone followup planned	24,962	3.6
Referred to other physician	20,071	2.9
Returned to referring physician	6,139	0.9
Admit to hospital	7,163	1.0
Other	15,536	2.2

Source: DeLozier, J. E. & Gagnon, R. O. *National Ambulatory Medical Care Survey: 1989 Summary.*
(Advance Data no 203.) Hyattsville, MD: National Center for Health Statistics, 1991.

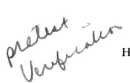

e. *Revising the data collection device*: Based on findings from above, revise the collection device. If revisions are substantial, repeat the pretest. Continue such repetition until you are satisfied with the instrument.

f. *Data collection conducted*: Here, data are collected according to a specified schedule, under common administration guidelines, at specified locations, and from a defined sample.

g. *Code preparation*: A code book should be prepared which lists the code used for each response to each question or statement presented on the data collection device. This is rather easy for closed-ended questions. For open-ended questions, it may be necessary to let the codes "emerge" from within the responses. To do this, read each open-ended response, searching for common themes. When found, record each separate theme and code those. Only one person should do this to help control for bias.

h. *Verification and editing*: Verification involves the re-administration of every n'th collection device, often every 20th, if at all possible. This is very important for interviews. When reading interview guides and/or responses, look to see if there was any tendency toward recording responses which seem inconsistent with what has already been said by the subject. When editing, look for consistency in responses and that "skip patterns" have been followed. Skip patterns are directions to skip a certain question or group of questions. For example, it is unlikely that a six year old would be attending high school. These activities should be on-going while the survey is being conducted, so corrections and/or changes can be made. If data are entered directly into a computer, as is commonly done in telephone interviews, a software program usually completes this step. Questionable responses can be quickly identified and corrected.

i. *Coding*: Once steps "g" and "h" have been completed, the data codes are readied for entry into the computer for processing. Data coding may be done directly on paper collection devices. Coding should be done only by those who are familiar with the survey's code book and who conducted verification and editing. If data are entered directly into a computer, this step is virtually eliminated.

j. *Entering data*: At this stage, data are entered into the computer for tabulation and analysis. The data entry operator should be thoroughly trained and closely supervised. Data related to a particular subject should be verified as in step "h" every 20th or so time.

k. *Tabulation and analysis*: Data are tabulated by a statistical software program. Usually, descriptive statistics are computed and printed. Aside from descriptive statistics, cross-tabulations are usually applied to data. A cross-tabulation combines responses to two or more questions or statements, such as sorting HIV positives by age or risk category. Additional statistical analyses may be conducted. Tabulation and analysis should be conducted by a person who is familiar with the purpose of the study, its subject matter, statistics, and the particular statistical processing program employed. If your study contains fewer than 30 or so cases (subjects) with less than 100 observations (data points), it may be easier to tabulate by hand. However, based on experience, the authors advise against such, if a computerized statistical processing program is available with the appropriate support. Additional tabulation is much easier and quicker by computerized means.

1. *Recording and reporting*: Each of the previous steps should be discussed in detail in the reporting document. Findings should be reported, interpreted, and discussed. It may be appropriate to include recommendations. If including recommendations, do so in a separate part of the report and be sure to present the rationale for each recommendation.

Data from studies conducted in accordance with these guidelines will probably be of high quality and, hence, usable. Be cautious about using data from studies which fail to follow this process or where the process used is unknown. For additional information, see *Survey Research Methods* by Babbie (1990) or *Mail and Telephone Surveys* by Dilman (1978).

HSR DESIGN CONSIDERATIONS

In planning and conducting survey research, there are other considerations requiring further discussion. These considerations include sampling, data collection, data analysis, and data reporting. Further, these considerations apply to descriptive demographic and epidemiologic studies.

Sampling: Introduction

Sampling is a very important consideration in research design. A sample is a subset (i.e., a small portion) drawn from a very precisely defined population. A sample (as well as a population) may be comprised of people, patient charts, organizations, animals, or any other object of interest. A sample is a device that allows us to conduct surveys (or other types of research) in a very manageable fashion. For example, suppose you wanted to do a survey of all hospital staff nurses in the United States. There are hundreds of thousands of nurses in that population. To make the survey process less expensive and easier to conduct, a sample of a few hundred hospital staff nurses could be drawn from that very large population.

A group, to be studied, is often referred to as a sampling frame. The construction of an accurate sampling frame for the hundreds of thousands of hospital staff nurses would take a very powerful computer, large budget, and much work and time. A sample frame this size would be subject to sampling error as people move, are promoted, leave nursing, enter nursing, and so on. Sampling error is the degree to which a sample's characteristics vary from those of the population from which the sample was drawn. To learn more about sampling error, see Welkowitz, Ewen, and Cohen (1991). If the sampling frame is small, and there are resources available (e.g., a desktop computer), the researcher should construct his or her own sampling frame to further reduce possible error or bias. Remember, a sample is only as good as its sampling frame. Once the sampling frame is constructed, the sample is ready to be drawn. There are two basic types of sampling: probability and nonprobability.

Probability sampling has been defined by Rubinson and Neutens (1987, p. 85) as, "those wherein the probability of selection [into a sample] of each respondent, or address, or even object, is known." For example, suppose there are one hundred addresses in a small town. Each address would have a 1 in 100 (i.e., 1%) chance of being included in a sample. The key advantages of probability sampling are: (a) error can be estimated and (b) a claim of sample representativeness of the population can be made. Generally, the smaller the sampling error, the more representative the sample is of the population; hence, the ability to generalize results beyond the sample, back to the larger population, is enhanced.

Nonprobability sampling was defined (Rubinson and Neutens, 1987, p. 90) as, "the probability that a person will be chosen is not known, with the result that a claim for representativeness of the population cannot be made." Sampling error is unknown and the ability to generalize beyond the sample is very limited, if not obviated. Nonprobability sampling is useful in pilot testing survey or interview forms. If the purpose of the study is not to generalize and if the population is very small (i.e., 100 or less) and if resources are limited, then a nonprobability sample may be useful.

While there are several strategies from which to choose, the sampling strategy selected should be appropriate for the reason the study is being conducted. Generally, it is preferred by experts that probability sampling be used in almost all studies, where possible. We will now briefly examine each of the above sampling strategies.

For your convenience, the various sampling strategies, as presented by Rubinson & Neutens (1987, pp. 85–91), are summarized and presented below:

Table 7.5   Sampling strategies

Probability	Nonprobability
Random	Convenience
Systematic	Quota
Stratified Random	Dimensional
Cluster or Area	Purposive
	Snowball

Sampling: Probability

Random sampling   This is the simplest form of probability sampling. Subjects are selected without bias or prior exclusion. Every subject has an equal chance of being included in the sample. Suppose you had four hundred clients in a primary prevention program targeting pregnant, low income women. A sample of 50 patient charts was to be audited every quarter to assess appropriateness and quality of care. Since random selection was desired, patient social security numbers could be printed on a page (sampling frame). The first three digits of the patient's social security number could be compared to a table of random numbers; the first 50 matching numbers would comprise the sample. A table of random numbers is a list of randomly printed numbers, with no relationship, on a page. Its use ensures that each of the 400 patients had an equal chance of being selected. Once the audit (also called monitoring) has been completed, the findings can be generalized back to the entire 400 patient population.

Systemic sampling   Rubinson and Neutens (1987, p. 86) have described this form of sampling as, "the selection of specific items in a series according to some predetermined sequence. The origin of the sequence must be controlled by chance [random]." Returning to our primary prevention project example, once the list of four hundred social security numbers was randomly printed, every fourth number could be selected up to the predetermined sample size of 50.

For the new researcher, a systematic sampling approach might be easier, provided a sampling frame can easily be constructed. If evidence of bias in the ordering is found, then the sampling frame needs to be redrawn or another sampling strategy employed. A systematic sampling approach could require the use of desktop computers or more powerful models, depending on the number of items in the sampling frame. To list thousands of addresses would require a computer.

Stratified random sampling   Rubinson and Neutens (1987, p. 86) have described this form of sampling as, "the population is broken down into nonoverlapping groups called strata, and then a simple random sample is extracted from each stratum." The objective is to "subdivide the population into smaller homogeneous groups in order to get a more accurate representation or to include parameters of special interest [e.g., disabled Hispanic persons] (p. 87)." Once a stratum or grouping has been formed, a simple random sample is drawn.

Returning to our example of hospital staff nurses, we could form three strata: urban/rural, male/female, and hospital size, with five categories (called levels). Each strata can have different levels (e.g., two or five, as in our example). The contribution of subjects to the sampling frame by each strata is determined. Percentages are calculated and then applied to the sample. Through application of simple random sampling, subjects are then enrolled in each of the sample's strata. The object is to have the same or similar percentage distribution of strata membership in the sample as in the population.

If applied carefully, great accuracy results. However, given the complicated process by which the sample is drawn, the possibility of error is increased. This sampling strategy is usually reserved for very large studies conducted by large corporations and governments. It is rarely applied in operations level HSR.

Cluster or area sampling   This sampling strategy is most useful when a sampling frame can not realistically be constructed as in our hospital staff nurse example. Rubinson and Neutens (1987, p. 89) outline an illustrative example of application which follows:

> If an investigator proposed to survey all public school health educators in the United States, a simple random sample would be impractical. In multistage cluster sampling the investigator can first randomly sample 20 of the 50 states. In the second stage, from a sampling frame that lists all counties within the 20 states, a random sample of 100 counties could be selected. Then, in the third stage, a random sample of 50 school districts could be drawn from all the school districts within the 100 counties. The fourth stage consists of random selection of 100 school health educators in the 50 school districts. The successive random sampling of states, counties, school districts, and finally health educators is relatively inexpensive and efficient.

As in stratified random sampling, cluster sampling is usually reserved for large studies. Cluster sampling is subject to the possibility of significant error, as it really is a sample of samples. The use of cluster sampling requires special expertise which should be sought if a sample is to be so constructed.

In operations level HSR, sample sizes tend to be rather small (a few hundred cases). The selection of either the simple random or systematic strategies is probably more one of personal choice than anything else. Based on experience, the authors prefer the simple random selection strategy, given its high degree of accuracy and relative ease with small sampling frames. Stratified random sampling and cluster sampling are rarely used in operations level HSR.

Sampling: <u>Nonprobability</u>

Convenience sampling   A convenience sample is composed of those subjects who are most convenient. For example, suppose we wanted to study prenatal patients. So, we developed a questionnaire and went into the health department's waiting room and surveyed all the prenatal patients present. We could report our findings; but, those findings would have little relevance beyond the group of patients which just happened to be in the waiting room at the time we surveyed.

This strategy almost always produces a sample which is not representative. While time and money are saved, the results are routinely dismissed. It is advisable to avoid conducting a study based on a convenience sample or using the results of one in your planning efforts.

Quota sampling This strategy is equivalent to stratified random sampling, except that subjects are not randomly selected. Once the quota of sample subjects is set for each strata, the researcher finds eligible subjects to fill each quota. The researcher should try to avoid bias in selecting subjects. A claim of representativeness is more difficult to support in quota sampling than in stratified random sampling because of increased sampling error.

Dimensional sampling In dimensional sampling, all the variables of interest (e.g., gender, race, age category, and HIV status) are specified. In the sample, at least one subject with each characteristic, and every possible combination, must be present. A small sample is drawn and each case is examined in detail. As in quota sampling, the researcher locates eligible subjects and should avoid bias in selection.

Purposive sampling The researcher selects those subjects who best meet the purpose of the study. This strategy does not rely on random selection (i.e., probability) but on the experience and judgment of the researcher. In the authors' opinion purposive sampling should only be employed by experienced researchers. This sampling strategy is routinely used in pilot testing survey and interview forms as well as in those instances where there is no need to generalize beyond the sample.

Snowball sampling In this sampling strategy, subjects possessing the desired characteristics are interviewed. These subjects suggest others possessing the same characteristics, who are in turn interviewed. This process continues until the desired sample size has been reached. Snowball sampling can become a probability strategy if simple random sampling is done at each stage. This strategy can be very useful in attempting to study hard to reach populations, such as IV drug users or other substance abusers.

Sampling: Sample Size

The determination of sample size can be a rather complex issue. In operations level HSR, we are more concerned with representativeness than sample size. However, sample size has a direct relationship to representativeness, as does random selection. Formula for calculating sample size are beyond the scope of this presentation. Further instructive reading may be found in Rubinson and Neutens (1987) and Welkowitz, Ewen, and Cohen (1991).

Sample size guidelines are difficult to formulate and subject to much debate. However, for statistical analysis, Welkowitz, Ewen, and Cohen (1991, p. 227) recommend samples of at least 25 to 30 subjects. Rubinson and Neutens (1987, p. 92) suggest a minimum of 100 cases in a sample, if that sample is to be subdivided, e.g., males and females, or white and nonwhite. Generally, the larger the sample, the less sampling error, and the greater representativeness of the sample. Again, the desirability of random selection of sample members can not be overstated.

Data Collection Methods: Introduction

Data may be purchased from research, marketing, and other such companies. Universities may sell data or make it available in special library collections or government document sections. Also, a significant source of data is the organization's management information system. If either purchasing or using data from other sources, be sure there is a statement about how those data were collected attached to the data report.

In those instances where it is necessary to collect your own data, there are a variety of collection mechanisms that may be employed. Select the method (or combination) that best suits the purpose of the study and the organization's capacity to successfully complete a study.

Some of the most common data collection methods are the questionnaire, interview, and document review (e.g., chart audit). All three methods have several assumptions in common, which are:

a. that the instrument containing questions or statements and the recording sheet(s) have been developed, peer reviewed, and thoroughly pilot tested prior to data collection;
b. that the researcher has sufficient knowledge, so as to ask the right questions or abstract the required data;
c. that the researcher will suspend his or her personal beliefs and judgments, so as not to bias subject responses or data;
d. that subjects will honestly answer questions, respond to statements, and not alter behavior so as to deceive study investigators; and
e. that data collection personnel have been thoroughly trained with respect to the purpose of the study, correct administration of the data collection device, and confidentiality issues.

These assumptions should be kept in mind when evaluating the quality of data produced by a study or in conducting your own. It is particularly important to ensure that these assumptions are addressed in reporting study results.

Data Collection Methods: Design Considerations

Each of the three data collection methods, referenced above, have several common design characteristics which include question types, guidelines for item (i.e., question or statement) construction, formatting and reproduction, item ordering, instructions, training, reliability, and validity.

Question types There are two types of questions: closed- and open-ended. Closed-ended questions present response options to the respondent. Open-ended questions allow the respondent to respond as he or she sees fit. Question 1 is closed-ended. Question 2 is open-ended.

1. What is your current age in years?
   a. 17 years or less   [   ]
   b. 18 years   [   ]
   c. 19 years   [   ]
   d. 20 years   [   ]
   e. 21 years   [   ]
   f. 22 or more years   [   ]
   g. Don't know   [   ]
   h. Refused   [   ]
2. What do you see as the most important human resource management issues facing healthcare managers today?

   _____

   _____

   _____

Closed-ended questions provide uniformity in responses, which makes data processing easier. Since response options are generated by the researcher, it is expected that the researcher has a very thorough understanding of the subject under investigation. The authors have found that conducting a preliminary survey with almost exclusively open-ended questions can be very helpful in framing closed-ended questions. When using closed-ended questions, the response options should be mutually exclusive and the list exhaustive.

Open-ended questions require coding by the researcher, provide for more expression opportunity for the respondent, and should be precisely phrased. When coding responses, be consistent. Irrespective of the type of data collection method chosen, all require that an instrument be developed and ready for use prior to the start of data collection.

Statements The most commonly used statement in survey research is the Likert Scale. Within this format, a statement is made. The respondent is asked to agree or disagree along a scale. Question 3 is an example:

3. I prefer to provide direct patient care rather than perform administrative duties.

Strongly Disagree	Disagree	Neutral	Agree	Strongly Agree
1	2	3	4	5

If using the Likert Scale, be very precise as to what the statement is addressing and avoid double negatives. For additional information, see *How To Measure Attitudes* by Henerson, Morris, and Fitz-Gibbon (1987).

Item construction guidelines   Babbie (1990, pp.129–131) has suggested several item construction guidelines. These are, as adapted: (a) make items clear, (b) avoid double-barreled questions [be careful when using "and" or "or"], (c) be sure the respondent is competent to answer, (d) items should be relevant, (e) short items are best, (f) avoid negative items, and (g) avoid biased items or terms. Make responding to the item as easy as possible. It is probably best to use a combination of open-ended and closed-ended questions as well as Likert Scale style statements.

Formatting and reproducing   Don't crowd the text on to a page. Make skip patterns (i.e., skipping some questions, as directed) as few and as simple as possible. Make the appearance of the instrument attractive. If using open-ended questions, give the respondent enough room to write the response. When reproducing the instrument, use high quality, sturdy paper. The instrument should be easy to read. There should be sharp contrast between print and page.

Item ordering   It is probably best to place the following items towards the end of the instrument: the most sensitive items, rather involved items, and demographic items. It is advisable to place a screening item first. The purpose of the screening item is to prevent respondents, who you really don't want to participate in the survey, from doing so. If you were surveying laboratory technologists, it is doubtful you would want the laboratory's clerk participating in the survey.

Instructions   Directions should be clear and simple. Give an example of how you want questions answered. The less effort a respondent has to expend, the better. Drawing a circle or placing a check in a blank are acceptable. Remember to advise respondents to be careful and make their response choice very clear.

Training   If data collection assistants are to be used, they should be thoroughly trained. Assistants may be utilized in all of the data collection methods presented, except the mail survey. The "typical" training module includes an orientation to the study, review of the data collection instrument, copious practice sessions, role playing, alternating roles, and at least two mock administrations involving the researcher or a supervisor. For direct administration surveys or document reviews, practice sessions may be fewer in number. However, for interviews, more intense practice sessions and role plays should be employed.

Reliability   As defined by Isaac and Michael (1981, p. 125), reliability "refers to the accuracy (consistency and stability) of measurement by a test." Unreliable (i.e., unstable) instruments often produce inaccurate or biased results. Reliability is estimated by application of statistical formula which produces a coefficient ranging from zero to one. The closer the co-efficient is to one, the more reliable the instrument is said to be. Because there are different types of reliability (e.g., internal consistency and test-retest), there are different types of coefficients.

If an instrument to be used in a study is purchased, it is a good idea to ask for evidence of reliability. Many surveys are conducted with locally developed instruments which are administered only once. If needed expertise is lacking, the researcher should at least do the following: (a) describe very clearly what is needed to be known; (b) develop and refine questions until there is no ambiguity in the item; (c) test the questions or statements with a sample similar to those who are to be studied; (d) ask the pilot test sample to suggest ways to improve the clarity of each item [give room on the instrument to do so]; (e) have the instrument reviewed by a jury of experts before and after each pilot test; (f) if scales (e.g., Likert type statements) are used, try to have ten or more statements; and (g) draw a sample which is as large as possible. While these suggestions are not intended to substitute for the determination of an instrument's reliability, they do provide useful guidance for ensuring some measure of reliability.

Validity   Isaac and Michael, (1981, p. 119) define face validity as, "on the face of it, appears to measure what it claims to measure." From a technical perspective, face validity is not a strong concept; but in survey research, face validity is of prime political importance. In survey research, we are also concerned with content validity. Validity can be assessed by using statistical formula. If purchasing an instrument, ask for evidence of validity. If you are developing an instrument locally and lack access to the needed expertise, follow the steps outlined in the discussion of reliability.

These are intended as general guidelines. A more detailed discussion is found in Babbie (1990).

Data Collection Methods: Questionnaires

Introduction   There are three mechanisms for administering questionnaires: direct administration, mail, and telephone. Only the mail survey does not require personal, face-to-face interaction between the subject (also called respondent) and the researcher.

In descriptive HSR, it has been the authors' experience that mail (traditional and electronic) and direct administration are the most common formal surveys conducted in the healthcare work environment. In community health studies, telephone and direct administration surveys (usually in the form of a household interview) are most common. Direct administration and telephone surveys tend to cost more than mail surveys due to expenses associated with training, supervising, and supporting human interviewers.

Direct administration   Direct administration, usually involves face-to-face inter-action between researcher and respondent. Accordingly, it is very important that the researcher does not engage in behavior which may affect how a subject responds. Dress and language should suit the survey purpose, administration site, and subjects. Those administering a questionnaire should be thoroughly trained and read from a prepared script when providing directions. Generally, the researcher should *not* read questions or statements to the respondent(s).

Administration practices should be consistent if the survey is administered by more than one person or in more than one location. In no case should questions or statements be explained or interpreted. If a respondent does not understand, slowly read the question or statement again. The administration site should be quiet, well lighted, comfortable, convenient, safe, and accessible. If at all possible, responses should be anonymous.

Mail surveys It is essential that mail surveys be thoroughly pilot tested prior to mailout. Errors in directions, skip patterns, sentence structure, or response options cannot be easily corrected once the questionnaire has been mailed.

Response rates increase with repeated contacts. According to McMillan and Schumacher (1984, p. 163–164), the first mailout (cover letter, questionnaire, and self-addressed stamped envelope) should generate a return rate of forty to sixty percent, while the first followup (reminder notices) should bring in ten to twenty percent more responses (returned questionnaires). A second followup (second reminder notice, questionnaire, and self-addressed stamped envelope) will probably bring in another five to ten percent. Response rates above sixty percent are considered very good. Acceptable response rates are between fifty and sixty percent (1984, p. 164). It has been the authors' experience that a third followup (reminder notice) will generate between five and ten percent additional responses.

A well constructed sampling frame will assist in generating a high response rate, as precision is increased. Questionnaires are less likely to be sent in error to inappropriate subjects. Suppose you were conducting a survey designed to assess nurses' attitudes towards computerized patient charting and several dozen computer sales associates (none of them nurses) were included in the sampling frame. It is likely that some of those sales associates would respond (thus contaminating results), but most would not. Because of an inaccurate sampling frame, the survey response rate would be lower than otherwise would have been expected.

The cover letter is very important in assuring a high response rate. The essential elements of a cover letter, as outlined by McMillan and Schumacher (1984, pp. 163–164), have been adapted and are presented below:

a. *Identify the purpose of the study and investigator.* Introduce the study and briefly describe its purpose. Clearly identify yourself (it is not necessary to list your name).

b. *Importance of the study.* This is your opportunity to briefly describe to the subject the contribution the study will make.

c. *Importance of the respondent*. In this paragraph, tell the respondent how important the response is to the study and that failure to participate will adversely affect the study and lead to incomplete results. Request cooperation at this point.

d. *Study endorsement*. Tell the respondent who has endorsed the study. It is probably best to avoid the use of individual names. Use titles and/or organization names. Be careful to have documented the endorsements claimed.

e. *Description of the questionnaire*. Briefly describe the questionnaire. Explain its essential elements. Tell the respondent about how long it should take to complete the instrument. Ask the respondent to complete and return the questionnaire as quickly as is convenient. Always give a deadline date.

f. *Assurance of confidentiality*. Point out that the subject's responses are anonymous or at least confidential. Whenever possible, participation should be voluntary and anonymous.

g. *Closing*. Give the respondent an opportunity to obtain a summary of the results, if appropriate. Always thank the respondent.

Sign the cover letter. The shorter the cover letter, the better, provided each of the above elements is adequately addressed. Be sure that the letter is clear and presentable, words have been spelled correctly, punctuation is correct, and grammatical rules have been followed.

Telephone surveys   Telephone surveys are routinely utilized in political polling, marketing research, and behavioral health risk factor surveillance systems. Since telephone surveys are very complicated and expensive to conduct, they should be conducted only by those who are specifically trained to do so. For more information, see *Telephone Survey Methods* by Lavrakas (1987) and/or *Survey Research by Telephone* (Frey, 1983).

Data Collection Methods: Interviews

Patton (1980, p. 206) has provided a convenient taxonomy for classifying interviews. The taxonomy is presented below:

"*Informal conversational interview*: Questions emerge from the immediate context and are asked in the natural course of things; there is no predetermination of question topics or wording.

Interview guide approach: Topics and issues to be covered are specified in advance. In outline form, interviewer decides sequence and wording of questions in the course of the interview.

Standardized open-ended interview: The exact wording and sequence of questions are determined in advance. All interviewees are asked the same basic questions in the same order.

Closed quantitative interviews: Questions and responses are determined in advance. Responses are fixed; respondent chooses from among these fixed responses."

As you can see, as the questions and responses become more structured, the role of the interviewer and the nature of the instrument change. It is recommended that if data are to be collected via an interview, rigorous training of interviewers be employed.

In the conversational interview, there may be a lack of consistency in how questions are asked (some topics may not even be addressed). Data analysis may be difficult due to a lack of standardized responses. An advantage of this approach is that the interview can be tailored to the interviewee's natural setting and circumstances. To conduct such an interview, a thorough knowledge of the circumstances surrounding the study and the interviewee's place within those circumstances is needed. Further, great skill is required. The authors advise that only trained, experienced researchers utilize the informal conversational interview approach. An example of such an approach is a counseling session.

In the interviewer guide approach, the role of the interviewer is to cover all topics listed in the schedule at some point within the interview. While the interview guide provides increased structure, it allows the interview to flow naturally. Comprehensiveness is more assured, but responses can become less natural. The loss of respondent flexibility may reduce the amount of relevant data collected. An application of this approach is a print or electronic journalist interviewing a subject. Interviewers should be specifically trained, by experienced persons, to apply this approach.

The role of the interviewer is less central when the standardized open-ended interview is conducted. Within this approach, the interviewer asks questions and the respondent answers. The interviewer records the response as stated. Thus, the interviewer can influence interviewee responses by the way questions are read or how the interviewer behaves. Data collection is standardized and analysis is made easier. Training and supervision are essential. Interview instruments composed of only open-ended questions are examples of this approach. Political polling commonly uses this approach.

When closed quantitative interviews are used, respondents must select from the response options available. Thus, relevant data may be lost or distorted. While the role of the interviewer is further reduced, the design of the instrument becomes even more critical. Data collection and analysis is rather simple. An example of this approach is an interview instrument composed of only closed-ended questions. This approach is routinely used in telephone surveys.

In the first two types of interviews (informal conversational interview and the interview guide), the role of the interviewer is primary. Depending on the interviewer's behavior, appearance, verbiage, body language, or other characteristics, responses have the potential for being influenced. In the last two types of interviews (standardized open-ended and closed quantitative interviews), the role of the interviewer is less central to that of the data collection instrument. It is clear that the interviewer must be very well trained, and the interview instrument must be well developed.

Many researchers employ a set of methods often referred to as qualitative in nature. Qualitative research relies heavily on observation and description, is concerned with process rather than simply outcomes, and analyzes data inductively. Rather than administering a survey and objectively computing responses, the qualitative researcher is more likely to observe an object of interest, maybe conduct a few interviews, and write copious notes (called narrative). Later, the qualitative researcher will immerse himself or herself in the narrative, looking for logical patterns. Data analysis and conclusions emerge from this immersion. While time and labor intensive, qualitative research methods can enrich many health services research projects. For more information see Bogdan and Biklen (1982) and Patton (1980).

Data Collection: Document Review

Abstracting data from patient charts, meeting minutes, employee records, statistical reports, or other document sources are rather common for the operations oriented health care manager. These documents may be located in medical or institutional libraries, medical records departments, departmental or personal files, as well as the business office.

Prior to abstracting data, the researcher should have: (a) ensured that there was a clear and present need for those data being sought; (b) located data source(s); (c) developed the requisite data collection form(s); (d) obtained the needed cooperation agreements, if other organizations are involved; (e) ensured that the appropriate informed consent(s) have been given and the necessary forms have been duly signed, if needed; and (f) ensured that no applicable laws or regulations will be violated because of the abstracting.

Abstracting is actually accessing secondary sources of data. A secondary data source is less desirable than a primary source; however, often secondary sources are all that is readily available or even exist. Therefore, the authenticity of secondary sources must be verified through whatever means available (e.g., a collaborating primary or secondary source). Usually, the more recent the secondary source, the easier is authentication. A good rule-of-thumb is to have at least two collaborating sources.

The data collection form should be very well organized with a location for recording each datum. The collection form should be designed by those knowledgeable about the subject and reviewed by an expert. Further, the collection form should be field tested and revised until it is acceptable. Abstractors should be trained and supervised.

Abstracting from medical records is very common. When doing such abstraction, be sure that you record only what you can read. If you are unable to read any portion of the chart, data from other sections of the chart may provide the needed clarification. Otherwise, ask for assistance. Don't guess or infer data.

Data Analysis

Once descriptive HSR (as well as demographic or epidemiologic) data have been collected, edited, coded, and tabulated, the analysis phase begins. To tabulate data, the researcher routinely applies descriptive statistics. The statistics and/or raw numbers are presented as narrative, tables, charts, and/or graphs. A variety of presentation techniques is recommended. The authors have presented a discussion of descriptive statistics and presentation techniques in Chapter 6 which is applicable.

Based upon their experience, the authors suggest that once data have been tabulated, the researcher put the data set aside for at least a few days. After the few days have passed, the researcher should review the data for consistency and to see if it makes sense. Once this has been done, the researcher begins the process of interpreting the data for the reader(s).

Data interpretation is aided by (a) a thorough knowledge and understanding of the subject matter; (b) a thorough review and discussion of the relevant, recent literature; (c) the aggressive use of peer review; and (d) the cogent blending of "a through c" in the discussion section of the reporting document. Data must be interpreted if they are to provide any meaningful guidance to planning and/or management efforts.

Data Reporting

The reader should be guided through the reporting document by the writer. Criteria for well written documents were presented in Chapter 4, as were resource suggestions. The authors cannot overstate the importance of well written documents.

There is no single model for organizing reporting documents. McMillan and Schumacher (1984, pp. 31–40) have presented an excellent discussion of the research article and its divisions. The authors suggest that this form of document organization is suitable for most reports of descriptive demographic, epidemiologic, and health services research. McMillan and Schumacher's model, as adapted, is presented and discussed below:

   a. *Abstract*: Within the abstract (also called executive summary), the study's subjects, methods, and salient points are summarized. The purpose of the abstract is to provide a reader with enough information so the reader may decide whether or not to read the document.

b. *Introduction*: In the introduction, the context of the study is set. This is usually done through a very brief summary of relevant literature. The introduction is rather general and is a "lead in" to the more specific purpose of the study, i.e., the question, problem, or issue addressed by the study.

c. *Statement of the problem*: The relevant question, problem, or issue is introduced and described. This description may include at least the following: (a) a thorough description of the question, problem, or issue; (b) clues that lead you to believe a question, problem, or issue exists; and (c) consequences of the problem, issue, or unanswered question to the institution, its personnel, or customers. Draw from the relevant literature.

d. *Review of relevant literature*: In this section of the report, the question, problem, or issue is analyzed in detail. This analysis may include at least the following: (a) why you believe the question, problem, or issue exists, (b) factors which support the existence of the question, problem, or issue, (c) factors which may hinder effective resolution of the question, problem, or issue, or the ability to capitalize on an opportunity, and (d) any other relevant information. This discussion should be based on theory and research drawn from the relevant literature.

e. *Methodology description*: In this part of the report, the methodology of the study is described. It is appropriate to describe how the survey process was followed by the present study and how each of the previous assumptions underlying the data collection options were addressed. The data collection instrument should be described as well as how data were analyzed. Reserve a copy of the instrument to an appendix.

f. *Results*: Here, the results of the present study are presented. The presentation should be straightforward and devoid of editorial comment. Keep tables, charts, graphs, and narrative as simple and as uncluttered as possible.

g. *Discussion*: In this section, the findings (results) are interpreted and related to the statement of the problem as well as the review of the relevant literature. Explain any unexpected results or problems in methodology. Usually, implications of the findings are included. If recommendations are made or conclusions are drawn, be sure to provide a rationale which is grounded in the study's findings and the relevant literature.

h. *References*: List all references cited in the document. Remember, references can be interviews, journal articles, memorandums, protocols, internal documents, or other relevant sources.

Many reports and journal articles will not follow this form of organization. However, most well written documents and/or articles will contain similar information.

It may be helpful to the reader to have an introductory paragraph which explains how the document is generally organized. The combined use of a "road map" paragraph with headings will help the writer "walk" the reader through the document.

Once the first draft of the report is written, set it aside for a few days. Review and revise the report, as needed. It is a good idea to have at least one or more peers read and critique the report. The importance of using correct grammar, spelling, and punctuation is obvious. For rather important reports, employ a proofreader and/or editor. A report's visual impact is tremendous. The visual impact sets a level of expectation and impression that even the most objective reader has a hard time shaking. While visual impact is important, most readers are not impressed by glitz. The substance must be present, as well.

SUMMARY

Health services research methods (i.e., surveys, interviews, and abstracting) provide relatively powerful, simple, inexpensive, and quick mechanisms to gather data which are to be used in health planning. For HSR data to be useful, it must be timely, verifiable, presented concisely, and presented without bias. HSR data may be found in reports, journal articles, and presentations at professional meetings.

The use of survey research methods is common. The "typical" survey is a set of 12 sequential steps. These steps are commencing the survey, survey design, construction of the collection device, pretesting the device, revising the data collection device, collection of data, code preparation, verification and editing, coding, entering data, tabulation and analysis, and recording and reporting. Surveys may be conducted over the telephone, in person, through the mail, or via computer. Usually a sample is drawn. Samples may be either probability or non-probability in design. Data collection methods include questionnaires, interviews and document reviews. Once the survey is completed, it should be reported. Such a report should include an abstract, an introduction, a statement of the problem, review of relevant literature, description of methodology, results presentation, discussion, and reference list.

REVIEW AND APPLICATION QUESTIONS

Directions. Read each question very carefully before selecting your answer. There is one correct answer for each question.

1. In order for health services research data to be useful on an operational level it must meet all of the following criteria EXCEPT:
   a. Be practical and timely
   b. Be applied to operational problems
   c. Be designed to produce data to identify problems
   d. The reporting level need not be considered when designing user reports.

2. Concerning Aday and Shortell's four dimensions of health services utilization each of the following statements is correct EXCEPT:
   a. Type refers to category of services rendered.
   b. Site refers to the standard reporting form to Medicare.
   c. Purpose refers to the reason care was sought.
   d. Time refers to contact, volume, & episodic patterns.

3. Typical applications of descriptive health services research include each of the following EXCEPT:
   a. Describing health services utilization
   b. Forecasting revenue needs
   c. Evaluating programs
   d. Resource allocation

4. During 1989, several observations regarding physician office visits were made. (Table 7.2). Each of the following statements is accurate EXCEPT (Hint, compare percents and rates):
   a. Persons 25–44 years made more office visits.
   b. Generally, the per person/per year rate increased with age.
   c. Males made more office visits than females, especially between 65–74 years.
   d. The visit rate was similar during the early years of life for males and females.

5. The survey research process consists of _____ phases.
   a. 8   c. 12
   b. 10   d. 14

6. The phase of the survey process where the sample is specified is the _____ phase.
   a. Commencing the survey   c. Verification
   b. Survey design   d. Coding

7. The definition, "subjects have an equal chance of being included in the sample" refers to _____ sampling.
   a. Probability   c. Population
   b. Nonprobability   d. Sample

8. The sampling strategy where "the selection of specific items in a series according to a predetermined sequence" refers to _____ sampling.
   a. Random   c. Cluster
   b. Stratified   d. Systematic

9. Of the following sampling strategies, which one is used routinely in pilot testing?
   a. Convenience sampling   c. Purposive sampling
   b. Quota sampling   d. Snowball sampling

10. The recommended lowest number of subjects to be used in a sample, which will undergo statistical analysis, is:
    - a. 20–24
    - b. 25–30
    - c. 31–34
    - d. 35–40

11. The question type where response options are presented to the subject is called:
    - a. Option selected
    - b. Likert Scale
    - c. Open-ended
    - d. Closed-ended

12. The definition, "refers to the accuracy of measurement by a test," refers to:
    - a. Reliability
    - b. Validity
    - c. Probability
    - d. Ordering

13. Which one of the following data collection methods requires face-to-face contact between subject and researcher?
    - a. Telephone
    - b. Mail
    - c. Direct administration
    - d. Both a & b

14. In surveys, the minimally acceptable response rate is:
    - a. 30–40 percent
    - b. 40–50 percent
    - c. 50–60 percent
    - d. 60–80 percent

15. The type of interview where, "questions emerge from the immediate context and are asked in the natural course of things," is _____ interviewing.
    - a. Informal conversational
    - b. Standardized open-ended
    - c. Interview guide
    - d. Closed quantitative

16. The process of "pulling data from existing records" is called _____.
    - a. Coding
    - b. Tabulating
    - c. Analysis
    - d. Abstracting

17. Concerning data reporting, each one of the following is considered accurate EXCEPT:
    - a. Report's visual impact is tremendous.
    - b. Introductory paragraph can be referred to as a roadmap.
    - c. There is a widely accepted model for reporting documents.
    - d. Data should be interpreted.

Case 1: Northwest County Health Department

Read the following health services research report and answer the following questions.

The Northwest County Public Health Department commissioned a study of the health care seeking behaviors of county residents (population 33,000). Northwest County (2,000 square miles) is located in the northern reaches of a western state. The region surrounding the county is rural, with the chief businesses being ranching, farming, and lumbering. There is a large retired population. The county seat's population is 10,000. There are three smaller towns in the county, with the largest being 1,200 in population. Average household income is $11,500, with the average household size being 3.6 persons. There is one private hospital in the county and one public health clinic, and both are located in the county seat. You have obtained a summary of the report with the following data:

Table 1 Sources of medical care, service payment, and provider location

Distribution of Services by Provider	%	Payment Source	%
Physician's Office	43.0	Private Insurance	34.9
Public Health Clinic	15.8	Own Money	34.2
Outpatient (Hosp.)	16.8	Medicare	25.0
Hospital ER	14.2	Medicaid	5.9
No Medical Care	10.2		

Source of Transportation	%	Provider Location	%
Private auto	64.0	County Seat	82.5
Friends	27.0	Other County Locations	15.4
None	9.0	Outside County	2.1

18. Which of the following statements *best* describes the status of health services delivery within Northwest County?
    a. County residents are either currently, or potentially, dependent upon public health insurance programs.
    b. County residents are currently heavily dependent upon public delivery of health services.
    c. Almost two-thirds of county residents appear to be able to meet appointments due to transportation access.
    d. Health services providers appear to be widely distributed within the county.

19. Which of the following statements *best* describes the status of health services delivery within Northwest County.
    a. At present, private physicians appear to provide a majority of the county's health services to residents.
    b. There is a potential for at least doubling public health services delivery, given the current distribution pattern.
    c. Almost all county residents seem to have geographical access to health service providers.
    d. Don't know

20. Which of the following statements *best* describes the residents of Northwest County?
    a. Rural, low income residents
    b. Rural, high income residents
    c. High population density
    d. Insufficient information

Case 2: Inpatient Length of Stay (LOS)

Read the following table and answer the questions:

Table 1 Inpatient average length of stay (in days) in short-stay hospitals, United States, 1989

Age and Region	Both	Male	Female
Total	6.5	7.0	6.1
Age			
<15	4.9	4.9	4.9
15–44	4.7	6.2	4.1
45–64	6.7	6.7	6.6
65 & over	8.9	8.6	9.1
Region			
Northeast	7.7	8.0	7.4
Midwest	6.4	6.9	6.1
South	6.3	6.9	5.9
West	5.4	6.2	4.9

Source: 1989 summary: National Hospital Discharge Survey. (Advance Data no 199.) Hyattsville, MD: National Center for Health Statistics, 1991.

21. In which region did males experience a longer LOS?
    a. Northeast   c. South
    b. Midwest   d. West

22. Which age cohort experienced the shortest LOS?
    a. <15 years   c. 45–64 years
    b. 15–44 years   d. 65 or more years

23. In which age cohort was there the greatest degree of difference between male and female LOS?
    a. <15 years   c. 45–64 years
    b. 15–44 years   d. 65 or more years

24. The greatest degree of difference in LOS is between which two regions?
    a. Northeast & Midwest   c. Midwest & South
    b. South & West   d. Northeast & West

DISCUSSION QUESTIONS

1. Select a survey research project you have recently worked on (or interview someone who has recently worked on one), and compare the process employed with the process outlined in this chapter. How do they compare?

2. Under what conditions would you select a nonrandomized as opposed to a random sample? What are the advantages of a random sample?

3. Compare and contrast the following data collection methods: questionnaires, interviews, and document reviews.

4. Compare and contrast quantitative and qualitative research methods.

8

Health Planning Methods: Budgeting

Chapter Ojectives:

1. Describe terms commonly used in budgeting.
2. Describe the construction of a line-item budget.

Schulz and Johnson (1990, p. 97) have described the relationship of budgeting to planning as "plans are developed to define what will be done and how the tasks will be accomplished. Budgets outline the resources dedicated to the achievement of the strategy [objective]—in other words, the costs that are expected to be incurred in the implementation of the [objective]."

Once a plan is implemented and becomes operational, funds are expended to support associated activities. The expenditure process should be closely monitored. Where unexpected or unacceptable variances occur, corrective managerial action should be taken, if warranted. Be sure to investigate any instance where actual expenditures exceed the projected amount.

We will examine two common types of expense budgets: line item and program. We will also consider revenue budgeting. There are more sophisticated types of budgets and financial analysis techniques, but they require far more discussion than can be accommodated here. The reader who is interested in such may find *Accounting: A Management Approach*, by Shillinglaw and Meyer (1983), or *Basic Accounting and Budgeting for Hospitals* by Pelfrey (1992) to be helpful.

THE LINE-ITEM BUDGET

Table 8.1 is an example of a line-item budget which organizes projected expenditures by line-item category. It is the simplest and most common form of budgeting used in operations planning. The budget presented in Table 8.1 will serve as the basis for much of the discussion presented within this chapter. Each line-item category will be fully developed and explained.

Table 8.1 Line item budget
Health Education Liaison Project, 1990

Line Item		Budgeted Amount
Personnel-Positions		$52,173.82
Administrator	$10,119.12	
Health Educator I	17,000.00	
Health Educator II	18,375.07	
Secretary I	6,679.63	
Personnel-Fringe Benefits		15,239.97
Administrator	2,955.80	
Health Educator I	4,965.70	
Health Educator II	5,367.35	
Secretary I	1,951.12	
Travel		7,825.00
Office Support		18,482.36
Office Equipment	9,350.00	
Office Furniture	3,825.00	
Office Supplies	1,760.00	
Office Space	1,151.16	
Office Utilities	0.00	
Telephone	2,396.20	
Educational Materials		9,880.63
Audiovisual Equipment	7,734.98	
Printed Materials	2,145.65	
Continuing Education		1,200.00
Other Costs		
Consultant Fees		1,000.00
	Total	$105,801.78

Basis: Hale, C. D. & Davis, R. C. (1985). *Health Education Liaison Program: Final Project Report.*

Staffing Pattern Costing

Staffing patterns and costs must be driven by the program's objectives, service targets, and activities. If resources are insufficient to staff the program, as needed, then either (a) obtain additional resources or (b) revise program objectives, service targets, and activities to ensure compatibility between resources and proposed actions.

Of course, program staffing and costing are sometimes difficult to determine. There are several techniques that can be used, including: (a) replicate the staffing patterns of similar programs; (b) have a consultant determine the program's staffing needs; (c) conduct a time and motion study, then base staffing patterns on the results; or (d) consult with peers and, based on collective training and experience, staff according to your best judgment. However, method "a" may fail to take into account your program's unique circumstances. For programs of modest size, "b" and "c" are probably too expensive. Method "d" probably comes closest to considering the program's unique circumstances (and ability to pay).

Consider the following staffing pattern and costing model. Before examining this model, remember the term "performance standard" which was introduced in Chapter 2. Take a few minutes to review it. The steps in the suggested staffing pattern and costing model are:

a. Review the service targets and activities to determine needed employee knowledge, skills, and licensure in order to compose a position description for each needed position. Be sure to specify the necessary education and experience most likely to ensure that the person filling each position has the required knowledge and skills. Be sure to name each position. It is most likely that your institution's human resources office will have position descriptions and titles that are commonly used;

b. Next, determine what should be a realistic performance standard for each position (Often, this is an estimate based on industry standards or the planner's expert judgment, as in our example);

c. Again, review the program's service targets and activities (given expected performance standards) to determine the number of positions and percentage of Full Time Equivalent (FTE) (i.e., percentage of a full-time position) that will be needed. One FTE = 100%. (Sometimes a program needs a position, but only a portion of an FTE);

d. Summarize what has been determined in the following manner to compute annual salary costs (Example based on Table 8.1):

Position	Salary Rate	FTE	Total Salary
1) Administrator	$30,664.00	33% $1/3$	$10,119.12
2) Health Educator I	17,000.00	100%	$17,000.00
3) Health Educator II	18,375.07	100%	$18,375.07
4) Secretary I	6,679.63	100%	$ 6,679.63
			$52,173.82

e. Next, compute the fringe benefit costs for each position. This can be done by consulting the institution's human resource office or payroll office. (Don't compute the costs paid by an employee for any benefit or income tax when computing the program's fringe benefit costs.) Summarize as follows:

Position Salary	FICA (7.61%)	Insurance (21%)	Worker's Comp. (0.6%)	Total
Administrator $10,221.33	$ 770.07	2,125.02	60.71	$ 2,955.80
Health Ed. I $17,000.00	$1,293.70	3,570.00	102.00	$ 4,965.70
Health Ed. II $18,375.07	$1,398.34	3,858.76	110.25	$ 5,367.35
Secretary I $ 6,679.63	$ 508.32	1,402.72	40.08	$ 1,951.12
				$15,239.97

There are a number of ways to compute insurance costs. In this example, we used the percent of total salary method. Consult with your institution's human resources office or payroll office. It's a good idea to have a peer review the work.

Travel Cost Determination

Travel costs routinely include mileage (usually a flat rate per mile), air fare, car rental, cab fare, meals, and other allowable transportation costs, (e.g., tolls and parking fees). Per diem means that the cost of room and board (meals) for a traveler are reimbursed at a specified daily rate regardless of actual costs.

Most institutions have very specific travel policies. A planner should have a copy of the institution's travel policies when projecting travel costs for a program. When computing projected travel costs, the following model may prove useful:

Position	[a]Mileage	$50/day Per Diem	Common Carrier	[b]Meals	Total
Administrator	$ 200.00	$200.00	$500.00	$100.00	$1,000.00
Health Ed. I	1,500.00	500.00	500.00	500.00	$3,000.00
Health Ed. II	2,000.00	600.00	500.00	600.00	$3,700.00
Secretary I	125.00	0.00	0.00	0.00	$ 125.00
					$7,825.00

[a]Mileage reimbursement rate is 20 cents per mile.
[b]Meals are reimbursed at $5.00 for breakfast, $10.00 for lunch and $15.00 for dinner.

It is fairly common for air fare, car rental, and cab fare to be included under the "common carrier" heading, with each listed separately. Parking fees and tolls are routinely included under the mileage heading but are listed separately and then added into the mileage reimbursement total.

Computing Office Support Costs

The office support line item typically includes office equipment, furniture (chairs, desks, tables, filing cabinets, etc.), supplies (staplers, rulers, paper, postage, and photocopy, etc.), space, utilities, and telephone. There is no magical formula for projecting these costs; however, there are some rules-of-thumb. Office equipment and furniture are usually "one time" expenses, i.e., a desk is purchased only once. In the next few pages, we will discuss some of those general principles.

Office equipment The selection of the right office equipment is an important decision. The following general guidelines may be helpful:

a. On paper, fully determine, for each position, the necessary equipment;
b. Obtain bids from three vendors with product and price guarantees (good for at least 90 days); and
c. Select the lowest acceptable bid, and base equipment cost projections on that bid.

The following explains how the line item (Table 8.1), office equipment, was derived:

Secretary	
1 Electric typewriter @ $750 ea.	$ 750.00
1 Personal computer @ $2500 ea.	2,500.00
1 Computer printer @ $1000 ea.	1,000.00
1 Integrated Software @ $600 ea.	600.00
	$4,850.00
Health Educators I & II	
1 Personal computer @ $2500 ea.	$2,500.00
1 Computer printer @ $1000 ea.	1,000.00
1 Statistical software @ $200 ea.	200.00
	$3,700.00
1 Service contract (1 year)	$ 800.00
	$9,350.00

It is a good idea to get a service contract for office equipment, but be sure not to duplicate warranty coverage. Remember, sometimes it is more cost effective to replace than repair broken equipment. It is also a good idea to get bids on service contracts; with a service contract, you are as interested in efficient and effective repair as price.

Office furniture   The following model may be helpful in projecting office furniture costs:

a. On paper, fully equip each position with the necessary furniture;
b. Obtain bids from three vendors with product and price guarantees (good for at least 90 days); and
c. Select the lowest acceptable bid and base furniture cost projections on that bid.

In Table 8.1, we see a line item for office furniture for $3,825, which was derived as follows:

Quantity	Description	Amount
3	Professional desks @ $275 ea.	$ 825.00
3	Professional desk chairs @ $150 ea.	450.00
1	Secretarial chair	200.00
1	Secretarial desk	250.00
1	6-person conference table	500.00
6	Conference table chairs @ $75 ea.	450.00
3	Guest chairs @ $50 ea.	150.00
4	4-drawer file cabinets @ $150 ea.	600.00
4	6' × 4' × 1' book cases @ $100 ea.	400.00
		$3,825.00

Office supplies   Once office equipment needs and program staffing patterns have been determined, one is ready to project office supply costs. The following model projects such costs:

a. The cost of supplying each professional and clerical position is determined (To determine the cost of supplying each position, count the number and cost of staplers, rulers, in-out baskets, hanging folders, file folder boxes, paper clip boxes, paper tablets, printer paper, printer ribbons, and other paper supplies which are likely to be used and then sum.);
b. These costs are summed; and

c. Add 10% of the total as an inflation factor, thus producing an office supply projection.

Avoid using sale prices. Base your projections on prices from a retail office supply company. Of course, office supplies should be purchased from a discount vendor if one is available. Office supply prices can fluctuate. By using this method, you are less likely to have underestimated the cost of office supplies.

For our example, the following office supply costs were estimated:

Administrator	$100.00	Photocopy	$ 500.00
Health Ed. I	100.00	Printer Paper	125.00
Health Ed. II	100.00	Ribbons	50.00
Secretary I	125.00	10%	160.00
Postage	500.00		$1,760.00

The project covered a large service area, hence the need for much postage. Since its objectives include both patient education and staff training, several training manuals needed to be produced, hence the $500.00 photocopy line item.

Office space and utilities   Projecting the cost of office space can be difficult. The cost of capital construction or improvement will not be considered. If the program planner's or manager's institution has guidelines or if industry trade standards exist, use those in determining how much space will be needed to conduct program activities. Otherwise, these general principles apply:

   a. Determine what are the program's personnel, equipment, furniture, and programmatic (e.g., storage, instructional, lab, conference room, examining rooms, etc.) needs;
   b. Estimate the square footage needed for each staff member and his/her equipment and furniture as well as programmatic needs;
   c. Determine an average price per square foot to rent office space in the area where the program is to be located (call four to five landlords; get a price quote; and then average); and
   d. Multiply the needed square footage by this average charge to compute an office space cost projection (Most landlords will negotiate rent. The more vacant office space in the area, the more likely the landlord will negotiate.).

It's a good idea to get a lease which clearly describes the terms and conditions. Have the lease reviewed by a lawyer. Try to negotiate with the landlord to include trash removal and janitorial service with the frequency and type of cleaning specified. Make sure parking space is available for staff and guests and that the office building and grounds are well lighted, secure, and reasonably safe. Remember that some landlords charge extra for parking; research this before any lease is signed.

Before signing any lease, research the cost of utilities, (i.e., electricity, gas, water, hot water, etc.). Consider very carefully before signing a lease that has utility costs included in the rent. Any cost savings gleaned from price reductions, rebates, or conservation would go to the landlord if utilities were included in the rent. On the other hand, if utilities were *not* included in the rent, utility increases would be the responsibility of the program. The easiest way to research utility costs is to ask to see copies of bills for the last 12 months. If these are not available, call the utility company for the information. They may be able to provide the needed data.

For the example from Table 8.1, we find the following:

Secretary (12′ × 12′) 144 sq. ft. × $3.62 =	$ 521.28
Health Ed. I & II (10′ × 12′) 120 sq. ft. × $3.62 =	434.40
Administrator (30% of 12′ × 15′) 54 sq. ft. × $3.62 =	195.48
	$1,151.16

The project, upon which the present example is based, was required to lease office space from its parent program. The lease included all utilities, janitorial services, and security.

Telephone A few suggestions are provided for the reader's consideration in purchasing telephone service: (a) if the program is to operate for two or three years, renting equipment may be less expensive; (b) take the option for telephone and wire maintenance, if possible; (c) each FTE position should have a separate telephone (and line, if possible); (d) have at least two lines (publish one, this leaves the second line free to return calls, etc.); (e) use touch-tone equipment, as it is easier to expand capabilities; and (f) take bids from long distance service vendors (remember, you are as interested in access and general service quality, as in price).

Returning to our example from Table 8.1, we see the following with respect to telephone service:

Secretary	
1 phone @ $3.00 & 1 line @ $13.95	= $ 16.95
Health Educator I	
1 phone @ $3.00 & 1 line @ $13.95	= $ 16.95
Health Educator II	
1 phone @ $3.00 & 1 line @ $13.95	= $ 16.95
FTC Long Distance Charge/line $3.50 × 3	= $ 10.50
Monthly Line & Equipment Charge	= $ 61.35
Estimated Long Distance Toll	= $ 120.00
Budgeted Monthly Telephone Costs	= $ 181.35
Annual Telephone Service Charges/$181.35 × 12 months	= $ 2,176.20
One-Time Installation Charges	= 120.00
Service Contract	= 100.00
	$ 2.396.20

Educational Materials

Projecting the cost of educational materials is much the same as for office equipment and supplies. Educational materials can come in the form of films, books, pamphlets, VCRs, 16 mm film projectors, contracted teaching personnel, or software [compact disks, CD ROM disks, and regular software programs] with the necessary computer equipment needing to be available.

Select the educational media and delivery technology that does the job, for the least price. One must also consider the audience for which the education is targeted as well as those persons delivering the education. For example, if much travel and equipment conveying is involved, less expensive and light educational media should be employed. If the audience is young, puppets could substitute for films. Whatever educational media are selected, it should be appropriate for the audience and the goal of the program as well as being logistically practical.

For the program on which our example is based (Table 8.1), it was decided to purchase continuous feed projectors which used 8 mm film. These projectors were light, durable, and affordable. One was purchased for each service delivery site (11) as were some patient education films. It was decided to purchase several thousand pamphlets on a variety of health topics (which were related to the 8 mm videos) for distribution to patients by health care providers. Thus, patients would receive patient education information from the film in the waiting room, the health care provider, and a pamphlet which was to be taken home. The following costs were projected:

11 Continuous feed projectors & four 8 mm films		
11 at $703.18 ea.	=	$7,734.98
Educational Pamphlets	=	2,145.65*
		$9,880.63

*The project jointly purchased a very large supply to obtain a volume discount.

Clinical Materials

While not included in Table 8.1, clinical materials often play an important role in assisting a program or project in achieving its objectives and, hence, goal(s). Clinical materials include both the cost of medical, dental, or laboratory equipment as well as the necessary supplies. Equipment set-up and maintenance costs should also be included. The selection of clinical materials requires specialized expertise. The planner should ensure that the clinical equipment and supplies to be purchased are sufficient to support the program's clinical service targets. Programs which do not require the purchase of clinical equipment or supplies need not include such as a budget line-item.

Continuing Education

Within the health professions, knowledge changes and evolves very rapidly, hence the need for continuing education. Many states require health professionals (e.g., nurses) to earn a specific number of continuing education units as a condition of licensure. Accordingly, health programs routinely budget continuing education monies for the development of their professional personnel. Some programs provide continuing education opportunities to their paraprofessional, clerical, and administrative personnel. In our example, the continuing education line item was defined to include only tuition, books, or fees. Travel associated with such continuing education was charged to the program's travel line item. Generally, each category of employee is budgeted a specific amount of continuing education monies. When an employee desires to attend a continuing education program, permission is requested and if granted, then the costs (i.e., tuition, books, or fees) are deducted from that employee's "account." For our example from Table 8.1, the following is noted:

Administrator	$ 300.00
Health Educator I	300.00
Health Educator II	300.00
Secretary	300.00
	$1,200.00

Other Costs

Miscellaneous costs include marketing, catering, insurance, speaker honorariums, consultant fees, physical plant modifications, or overhead costs. Sometimes a funding agency will allow a funded program or project to bill it for "overhead costs," which are referred to as indirect costs. Indirect costs could include capital, administrative, accounting, and other support costs incurred by an institution that sponsors the funded program, such as a university that has a department which received a grant to provide material and child health services. Usually, indirect costs, which may vary considerably, are billable as a percent of the total program budget. Be sure to find out whether or not indirect costs are allowable when seeking funding for a proposed program through a foundation or a level of government.

Budget Justification Statement

Program and/or project budgets are generally presented in two parts: (a) the line-item budget, as in Table 8.1, and (b) a budget justification statement, keyed to each line-item, which briefly explains the rationale for it. Detailed explanations should be reserved to an appendix.

THE PROGRAM BUDGET

A more sophisticated type of budget used in operations planning is called a program budget. In a program budget, costs are distributed, along line-items, across specific programs.

Fictional Home Health, Inc., Table 8.2, provides skilled nursing services through its Alpha program and semi-skilled services through its Omega program. Both programs were administered by an executive director, whose $50,000 salary, including fringe benefits, was divided equally between both programs. Alpha program employs one administrator, two secretaries, and six registered nurses (RNs).

Omega program employs one administrator, one secretary, two supervising RNs, and eight Certified Nursing Assistants (CNAs). One RN provides quality control services for each program. The salary is divided between both programs. The combined budget for Fictional Home Health, Inc., is $816,800.

THE REVENUE BUDGET

There are instances where the funds needed to support a plan must be generated from the sale of goods or services produced once a plan has been implemented. Thus, an important

Table 8.2 Program budget for Fictional Home Health, Inc.

Line Item	Program Alpha	Program Omega
Executive Director[a]	25,000.00	25,000.00
Program Personnel[a]	*$298,000.00*	*$248,000.00*
Administrators (2)	40,000.00	40,000.00
Skilled (8 RNs)	210,000.00	70,000.00
Non-Skilled (8 CNAs)	0.00	104,000.00
Secretaries (3)	28,000.00	14,000.00
Quality Control (1 RN)	20,000.00	20,000.00
Travel	*75,000.00*	*100,000.00*
Office Support	*16,900.00*	*19,250.00*
Office Supplies	5,000.00	7,500.00
Office Space	6,500.00	6,000.00
Telephone	1,400.00	1,750.00
Computer Services	4,000.00	4,000.00
Educational Materials	*3,500.00*	*1,400.00*
Audiovisual Equipment	1,500.00	500.00
Printed Materials	2,000.00	900.00
Continuing Education	*2,375.00*	*2,375.00*
Administrative CE	500.00	500.00
Nursing CE ($300 ea.)	1,800.00	600.00
CNA ($150.00 ea.)	0.00	1,200.00
Quality Control	75.00	75.00
Total	$420,775.00	$396,025.00

[a]Includes fringe benefits

part of budget development is a forecast of expected revenue. This type of budget is called a revenue budget. Robbins (1991, p. 254) defines a revenue budget as, "a budget that projects future sales."

To estimate future sales, the demand for an organization's goods and/or services must be made (called forecasting). Once future revenue has been forecast, it may become necessary to adjust a plan's goal(s), objectives, service targets, and activities, upwards or downwards, given projected revenue. This adjustment leads to balanced expense and revenue budgets.

Developing a revenue budget can be a very complicated process. Many institutions have a specialist in their finance or business office who can provide assistance. These specialists should be consulted. If an in-house consultant is not available, it is strongly recommended that an outside consultant be retained.

SUMMARY

As you can see, while building a budget is a detailed, laborious process, it is essential. In some instances, a program's planned objectives, services targets, and activities may have to be scaled down given financial realities. Just as objectives, service targets, and activities are plans for action, a budget is a plan for the financial expenditures to support those actions.

Three types of budgets were presented: line-item, program, and revenue. A model for constructing a line-item budget was outlined and fully developed. A budget justification should be submitted with a budget.

REVIEW QUESTIONS

Directions. Read each question very carefully before selecting your answer. There is one correct answer for each question.

1. Budgets which organize expenditures by resource input categories are called _____ budgets.
   a. Revenue   c. Line-item
   b. Strategic business unit   d. Performance

2. Budgets in which costs are distributed along input categories across specific programs are called _____ budgets.
   a. Strategic business unit   c. Performance
   b. Line-item   d. Program

3. Which one of the following staffing pattern models comes closest to considering a program's unique staffing needs and is most realistic for modest sized programs to use?

    a. Replicate the staffing patterns of similar programs.
    b. Engage a consultant to determine the program's staffing needs.
    c. Conduct a time and motion study and then staff accordingly.
    d. Given training and experience, staff based on your and peer's best judgment.

4. The portion of a budget which explains the rationale for various expenditures is called:
    a. Budget statement   c. Budget report
    b. Budget justification   d. Budget summary   133

5. Documents which outline the resources dedicated to the achievement of a program's objectives are called:
    a. SBU   c. Budgets
    b. Operations reports   d. Expenditure reports

6. Expenditures for such items as per diem and common carrier comprise which category?
    a. Personnel   c. Office supplies   p 126
    b. Continuing education   d. Travel

7. Concerning the construction of an educational materials category, all of the following statements are accurate EXCEPT:
    a. Selected educational media should be appropriate for the program's purpose and objectives.
    b. The price of educational media should not be a consideration in selection.
    c. The projection of educational materials expenses is similar to those of office supplies.
    d. In some instances, computer software can be considered educational media.

    P 131

8. Professional development expenditures (e.g., seminar fees) would be included in which category?
    a. Educational materials   c. Continuing education
    b. Clinical materials   d. Travel   132

9. Office supply costs can be projected after _____ and _____ have been projected.
    a. Travel and staffing
    b. Office equipment and office furniture
    c. Office furniture and staffing
    d. Office equipment and staffing   128

10. Worker's Compensation insurance costs are included in which one of the following categories?
    a. Personnel   c. Other
    b. Fringe benefits   d. Office supplies

DISCUSSION QUESTIONS

1. Explain the relationship between budgeting and health program planning.

2. Explain the difference between line-item, program, and revenue budgets.

3. Why is it important to investigate variances between the amount budgeted and the amount expended?

4. For the goal, objectives, service targets, and activities developed in chapter two, prepare a budget, including a budget justification statement.

9

Health Planning Methods: Implementation Strategies

Chapter Objectives:

1. Describe three program implementation strategies.
2. Define 12 OD intervention strategies.

Once a health plan has been developed, it then needs to be implemented. The implementation process can range from "very easy" to "very difficult." In the vast majority of very difficult instances, health plan implementation can be facilitated through the use of techniques and processes developed by a discipline known as organization development (OD). A knowledge of negotiation and marketing techniques will also aid plan implementation.

Within this chapter, we will examine: (a) the impact of change within organizations; (b) organization development, including processes and commonly utilized OD techniques; (c) negotiation; and (d) marketing. Our purpose is to acquaint you with the contributions that each of these bodies of knowledge can make to efficient and effective plan implementation.

THE IMPACT OF CHANGE

The plans which an organization develops for implementation will hopefully have involved those who will be most affected by the changes to be introduced. In actual practice, most organizations that must implement far reaching plans find considerable reluctance among employees to accept the proposed changes. This is true even if they participated in the planning process that led to the changes. However, resistance is reduced if those who are affected by a plan's implementation have participated in a plan's development.

There is a significant difference in writing a plan and feeling its impact. This is because change leads to uncertainty. Current methods lead to predictable results, and employees have learned to expect those results. Change, if significant, may lead to major shifts in established income, status, and power relationships among members of both the formal and informal organization. Longstanding friendships and working relationships may be disrupted. Because of the extensive and personal impact that change brings to employees, a perceptive manager will study all of the systems at work within the organization and develop effective methods for implementing change.

A system is an arrangement of individual, interrelated elements which when combined form an organized whole. Within an organization, there are many individual systems (e.g., departments) which form the whole organization.

There are formal, structural systems, such as those represented by the organizational chart, that identify the formal arrangement of various departments and positions. There are also behavioral systems (formal and informal) that are represented by the formal interactions between incumbents of various positions within the formal structural system (e.g., the second shift supervisor who reports to the laboratory director). In addition to the formal behavioral system, there exists the informal organization (e.g., interpersonal relationships based on social or technical interaction or those which grow out of a mutual respect), which is important to working relationships throughout the whole organization.

Knowledge of all the various systems in operation within an organization is desirable for an identification of problem areas and the means to eliminate the problem(s). This might be represented by the following situation:

A and B are directors of two divisions. C is a subordinate of B (formal structural system). C needs to know the plans on a project of A. The formal procedures require C to submit a request through B who, in turn, will contact A for the information. However, this might cause alarm since A is very sensitive about this project and would want additional clarification of the need (formal behavioral structure). Therefore, C asks the division's secretary to get the plans for him from A's secretary, who is a close friend and lunch companion (informal system).

Implementing a plan which requires change in formal organizational structure is usually less difficult than implementing a plan which requires change in the behavioral system or in the informal organization.

ORGANIZATION DEVELOPMENT: AN INTRODUCTION _____

In recent years, there has been much research and writing on the very difficult process of bringing about change within organizations. As a result, a special field of management has evolved that brings together management theory and the application of behavioral science. The field is generally referred to as organization development (OD). An accepted definition of OD follows (Rush, 1974, p. 32):

> "Organization Development is a planned, managed, systematic process to change the culture, systems and behavior of an organization, in order to improve the organization's effectiveness in solving its problems and achieving its objectives."

This is a very broad concept. Changing organizational culture will effect changes in value systems and the basic attitudes of employees. Changes in an institution's systems will impact the organization's structure and policy decisions. Changes in behavior imply long-term change which requires extensive time and significant resources. Plans that are very local in nature (i.e., departmental) may be just as difficult to implement as plans which affect the whole organization.

Change Agent Role

The typical planner or manager may not have the experience or training to accomplish organization development objectives in a complex situation. Therefore, there has developed within this management practice a specially trained consultant who intervenes on behalf of management in the organization. This person is usually referred to as a change agent. The experience of many executives has led them to believe that an external change agent may be most helpful in effecting the implementation of plans for change. Such an individual is not a long-term employee of the institution and, thus, can be viewed as having no personal stake in the outcomes which result from changes in values, behavior, policy, and structure throughout the organization. If an outside consultant is not required, a senior manager or a designated representative will act as an internal change agent.

The change agent is a catalyst to bring about change with the least possible disruption to the firm. The change agent is a facilitator who intervenes on behalf of management to insure acceptance and support for needed change. The change agent is also a professional resource who will build bridges between the behavioral systems and the structural systems within the organization. The change agent should have the training and education that will permit quick recognition of the forces at work in given situations.

For plans which will probably cause only minor disruption of established systems, the change agent may find that informing those affected as to why a plan needs to be implemented and then enlisting the assistance of those affected may be sufficient action to enable smooth plan implementation. In some cases, an exertion of managerial authority, in a skillful and concerned manner, will be sufficient to effectively implement a plan. If an OD consultant is needed to implement a plan that has been developed, refer to Chapter 3 for consultant selection guidelines.

Stages of Organization Development

Organization development may be viewed as a series of steps to be taken by a change agent. This is true whether the agent is an internal employee or a professional consultant from outside the institution. These steps may vary, but are usually followed in at least an informal way. These steps are:

a. Recognition of a need for change and establishment of client/change agent relationship;
b. Development of rapport between change agent and client group;
c. Collection of data for developing information about possible problems:
d. Diagnosis of problem situations;
e. Intervention through techniques to effect desired change that will resolve problem situations;
f. Assessment of the results of interventions to determine that OD objectives have been met; and
g. Stabilization of the new programs and termination of the client/change agent relationship.

Recognition of Need for Change   Often, the recognition of the need for change is an outcome of the strategic or operational planning processes which have resulted in a new plan that is to be implemented. The implementation process may identify the need for a consultant to bring about an orderly transition to changed systems, thus the introduction of a change agent.

In other cases, an organization may have reached a point of stagnation that causes management to seek a fresh approach to problem situations. The top management official would, in either case, initiate action to establish the client/change agent contract. The success of the change agent will depend on the active support and backing of the top manager.

Development of Good Rapport   The development of good rapport between the change agent and the members of the organization is essential in the OD process. Trust and the willingness to express personal beliefs and values by institutional members are important if the change agent is to get to the root of problem situations. Many intervention techniques, particularly in behavioral systems, require organizational members to reveal information which must be held in confidence by the change agent. If such information was not held in confidence, sanctions against individuals and failure of the OD process could result. Therefore, the change agent must create open communication and a relationship that guarantees total trust.

Data Collection and Problem Diagnosis   The diagnosis of problem situations requires the ability to cut through symptoms to get to the root causes of elements that inhibit plan implementation. Interviews, surveys, direct observation, and role playing will provide data for analysis. This phase of the process must be carefully managed to control for contamination factors, which inevitably affect data collection (See Rubinson & Neutens, 1987). Costs, time availability, validity and reliability considerations must be weighed in the light of the trade-off between methodological purity and practical logistics.

Intervention Techniques   The interventions selected by the change agent will be based on his experience, training, and the problem areas that need attention. Gibson, Ivancevich, and Donnelly (1988, pp. 724–725) provide a useful framework for analyzing these situations. They suggest that an OD program contains a series of levels or targets, which may be placed on a continuum ranging from organizational structure to individual-group behavior. The depth of interventions needed to change organizational structure are quite low. Those at the other extreme, where the behavior of individuals and groups are to be affected, require much greater depth of intervention and probably the employment of an external OD consultant.

An in-depth review of intervention strategies is not possible here. However, it may be useful to list some of the strategies. Many are discussed in undergraduate business administration courses. Other interventions require thorough study and extensive training if they are to be used effectively. For more information, see *Organization Development* by Robey and Altman (1982), *Organization Theory: Structure, Design, and Applications* (3rd ed.) by Robbins (1990), or *An Experimental Approach to Organization Development* by Harvey and Brown (1992).

Interventions designed to change organizational structure include: job enrichment, decentralization, matrix organization design, program evaluation review techniques (PERT), management by objective (MBO), sociotechnical design theory, and System 4 management. Behavioral change interventions typically include transactional analysis, laboratory training techniques, the managerial grid, team building, and the Johari Window. (See Appendix 9.A.)

Assessment of Results   After the organization has implemented its plans and the employees have evaluated their personal and inter-group relationships in light of the implemented plan, the evaluation process will determine if the changes introduced will result in a more effective organization. The problems diagnosed in an earlier stage should be solved. Improvements then need to become stabilized as the normal mode of operation.

Stabilization and Termination   The change agent is concerned with the changes becoming institutionalized. An effective change agent will have helped management incorporate a means of continued analysis and renewal of the entire system, such as a management information system. At this point, the change agent should be prepared to disengage from the project and leave the organization or, if an internal change agent, return to normal duties. This is often not an easy process. The consultant has probably become a major figure within the organization. Therefore, the consultant should gradually withdraw. Continued contact to clarify evolving situations and availability for crisis involvement will assist the termination process.

Effectiveness of Organization Development

There are many approaches to bringing about the acceptance of change. OD is a process that has been used extensively since the 1950s. There have been many successes and some significant failures. The use of a number of intervention techniques has proven more successful than the use of a singular intervention. The proper character, ability, and motivation of the change agent are important to success. A planner or manager who knows that he or she will face obstacles in introducing change to his or her institution would be well advised, as a minimum, to study the OD process and use those aspects that will help bring about acceptance to change. Of course, the behavioral interventions that demand a knowledge and awareness of personal psychology and intra-group training should best be left to the professional in that field.

EFFECTIVE NEGOTIATING

Winning support for plans to be implemented, convincing colleagues to accept proposals for forthcoming plans, and being an effective facilitator in an internal change agent role requires important skills that a good manager must develop. Being right is insufficient. Having the authority to direct actions is insufficient. The careful development of negotiating skills is necessary if the plans are to be implemented successfully.

Learning to understand the motives of other people, why they act as they do, and knowing how to turn a potential confrontation into a win-win situation is an important step in the development of leadership ability. It is not an easy lesson for most managers. In fact, the majority of managers never develop the ability to effectively and smoothly move the situation to the outcome or to the point that they wish it to be and, at the same time, have all of their colleagues support the decisions made.

One of the most perceptive pioneers in the field of management was Mary Parker Follett. She lectured to groups of business leaders in the United States and England during the early part of this century. A collection of her most important lectures has been published in a book entitled *Dynamic Administration: The Collected Papers of Mary Parker Follett* by Fox and Urwick (1982). The introduction to this book and Mary Follett's lectures on *Constructive Conflict* and *The Giving of Orders* provide an insightful study of effective negotiating. All students of management are encouraged to read this work.

Effective Negotiation: Integration

Miss Follett speaks of an "integration," which she defines as "the harmonious marriage of difference" (Fox and Urwick, 1982, p. xxv). She refers to integration as the "basic law of life" (1982, p. 36). All participants come to a situation with different ideas. They then participate in an evolving reciprocal relationship that considers all the factors in a situation (1982, p. xxvi). The result is a new situation where all parties win, where *consensus* is reached. The key word is consensus.

Miss Follett states that there are three ways to deal with conflict: "domination," where the will of one person is forced on another; "compromise," where one or both parties to the discussion must give up something; and "integration" (Fox and Urwick, 1982, p. 2). Integration means invention of new solutions and the realization that neither party must give up a portion or all of what they want. That would be compromise, a result that will always be less than satisfactory to all parties. Yet compromise is the most often heard word when people with different views must resolve a conflict.

Miss Follett gave an oft quoted (Fox and Urwick 1982, p. 3) illustration of what she means by integration:

> "In the Harvard Library one day, in one of the smaller rooms, someone wanted the window open. I wanted it shut. We opened the window in the next room, where no one was sitting. This was not a compromise because there was no curtailing of desire; we both got what we really wanted. For I did not want a closed room, I simply did not want a north wind to blow directly on me; likewise the other occupant did not want that particular window open, he merely wanted more air in the room."

Effective negotiation means that compromise is *not* the goal. The goal is for a solution that satisfies all parties. The process of conflict resolution calls for all those involved to focus on the problem situation. This is difficult because the people involved have strong feelings, are sometimes emotionally involved, and, having taken a position, are afraid of losing face if they change their position.

Negotiation Levels

There are always two levels of social interaction when groups or individuals enter into negotiation. The first level is the process of interaction between the individuals themselves. It is affected by past interaction or reputation. Have they opposed each other on other issues? Do the participants mistrust the motives of the other? Are they afraid they will be trapped in an unacceptable position? There must be a conscious awareness and controlled expression exercised in the discussions on the person-to-person level. The second level, and it affects both groups in the negotiations, is the interaction between each group and the situation. Why did the two groups come together? They want to solve a problem or arrive at an acceptable agreement on some matter. This fact gives both parties the opportunity to conduct the negotiations on a higher level of interaction. It permits the participants to direct their attention to the reason for discussion and avoid the problems of personal interaction.

The Law of the Situation

Mary Follett referred to the "law of the situation" (Fox and Urwick, 1982, p. 29), meaning that interaction should be depersonalized and all those involved should direct their attention to the situation.

Focusing on the situation at hand is difficult, particularly if others are attacking an individual on a personal level. Self-discipline is necessary. Constantly evaluating what is being said by others and planning for a response directed toward the situation is a difficult task.

There are a number of techniques that may be used to redirect the attention of the groups to the real purpose of a discussion. If the discussion strays from the subject, ask a question of the other group that forces an answer related to the subject. A very simple example would be to ask how a particular comment impacts on the situation. One of the best responses to personal attack, or to an extreme position, is no response at all! Silence on one's part becomes uncomfortable for the other side. It implies a termination of the discussion. It implies that the comment is unworthy of an answer. The other group will very likely interrupt the silence with a modified position in order to elicit a reply and further the discussion.

Negotiation in Meetings

Negotiation is not always two groups of people talking across a table in a formal discussion. Negotiation is involved in nearly all meetings. It is involved in many managerial leadership activities. Consider how a manager gives orders to staff, counsels subordinates, and informs them of their performance appraisal.

Following is a list of comments that pertain to effective negotiation. Consider them and evaluate your personal style of negotiation.

- Keep cool.
- Search for the underlying problem. Don't just evaluate symptoms.
- Don't be pressured or react to emotional threats.
- Bring differences into the open.
- Insist on fairness to all involved.
- Analyze the situation and consider alternative courses of action.
- Be truthful in expressing interests and opinions.

- Look to the future, don't dwell on the past.
- Be a good listener, try to get to the substance of the comments.
- Avoid confrontations.
- Focus on problems, not people.
- Invite response and criticisms of your position.

Summary

Life itself is a series of changes that result from interactions with others. Important decisions result from a search for a win-win situation with others. Interactions between parents and children or husband and wife frequently require negotiation between the participants. Adversarial relationships are generally unproductive in business as well as in the family. Although competition and winning have been ingrained in most Americans through the economic system and the prevalence of sports in our society, there is no reason to carry the competition into all of our activities.

An outstanding short book on negotiating skills is *Getting to YES, Negotiating Agreement Without Giving In*, by Fisher and Ury (1983). It is highly recommended for those who wish to read additional material on the subject.

MARKETING THE PLAN

Another essential step in planning activities comes about once one has created a new product or service to be offered by the organization. If the organization contains a marketing department, it would be appropriate for those specifically educated in marketing or practicing marketing responsibilities to create, in consultation with the product or service originator, a marketing plan.

It is possible that an annual institutional marketing plan (one that considers the entire health care organization) already exists. If such a generic marketing plan exists, a supplemental marketing plan to specifically market the new product or service should be created. In the absence of a general marketing plan, a product or service specific marketing plan should be created.

There are numerous books available to explain in detail the creation of product or service specific marketing plans, such as Cohen (1991, pp. 44–65) or Kotler and Armstrong (1990). The discussion that follows is an introduction to the process of creating a marketing plan.

Experts in preparing marketing plans agree that marketing plans for specific products or services should contain the following sections (although sections may appear under slightly different titles):

Executive Summary
Environmental Analysis
The Core Marketing Plan

If your plan includes a comprehensive marketing element (plan) for a product or service to be offered to the public, place the marketing plan in an appendix or submit it as a separate document. Regardless, briefly summarize the key points in the project description section of the planning document.

Executive Summary

The Executive Summary provides management with enough information to readily understand the goal(s) and recommendation(s). This summary should describe what needs to be done; how much money and other resources are required; who are the principal participants; and the specific financial measurements, such as return on investment or number of patients recruited, that might be anticipated.

There are planners who dismiss the Executive Summary as a minor component of the plan. However, seasoned planners will state that busy executives frequently rely on the Executive Summary to determine whether or not the ideas or recommendations, contained in the plan, are meritorious and deserve further consideration. Very few marketing plans are read word-for-word, cover-to-cover by busy executives; however, almost every executive will read the Executive Summary. You might conduct a self-audit to detemine if your writing skills enable you to prepare a convincing Executive Summary that is only two to three pages in length. If not, a technical writing class might be helpful.

Environmental Analysis

Situation Analysis   This section, frequently referred to as the current marketing situation, should describe the macroenvironment and task environment *into which the product or service will be introduced*. In the macroenvironment section, describe the prevailing economic conditions; demographics; political, legal, technological, social, and cultural factors which may exert influence on the development and introduction of the product or service. This discussion is fairly general and serves to set the context for the very specific discussion presented in the task environment section of the situation analysis.

In the task environment section, discuss: (a) the organization (What are its experiences in the market? What other related products are offered? Who are the suppliers? What are the financial and human resources? What position is maintained in the market?), (b) the competition (Who are they? What are their products and services? Who are their suppliers? What are their strengths and weaknesses?), (c) financial considerations (What is the availability or nonavailability of funds? What return on investment can be expected? What is the cost of implementing the marketing plan?), (d) the impact of the media (Are publicity conditions favorable to offer the new product or service?), (e) any special interests (Are there any political pressure groups that will affect the introduction of the product or service?), (f) governmental influences (Is there any pending regulation that will harm or help introduction of the new product or service?), and (g) legal aspects (Are there any laws in place or pending that will affect product introduction?).

Strengths, Weaknesses, Opportunities and Threats (SWOT) An internal assessment of the organization is presented in this section. It will be helpful to anticipate internal organizational strengths and weaknesses which may impact the organization *as the new product or service is introduced into the marketplace.* For example, has the facility been recognized for its sustained delivery of superior quality services (strength)? Does the facility have minimal experience with the product or service about to be introduced (a weakness)?

Once strengths and weaknesses have been identified, they should be prioritized for the likelihood of each occurring. Further, their most probable impact (positive or negative) should be forecast. This enables a preparation of options, in advance, to counter possible negative impacts that result from weaknesses or to capitalize on opportunities resulting from strengths.

An analysis of the external environment should reveal the opportunities and threats related to the new product or service as it is introduced. For example, is there a need for the product or service that is not currently being met in the marketplace (an opportunity)? Does the competition have the ability to enter the target market with a similar product or service soon after product introduction (a threat)?

Once external opportunities and threats have been anticipated, assign each opportunity a probability of occurring. This is done to identify which ones provide the best chance of achieving or improving the organization's competitive advantage with the new product or service. These probabilities will also help justify the risk involved with each opportunity. Threats should then be assessed for their probable impact during product or service introduction. Strategies should be developed to counter the probable impact of each threat.

The Core Marketing Plan

Goals and Objectives Having analyzed the strengths, weaknesses, oportunities, and threats, the planner should establish the goals and objectives to be achieved during the life of the marketing plan. Next, consider the issues that will affect these goals and objectives.

A goal, for example, may be to increase market share with the new product or service by four percent this calendar year. An objective may be to achieve one percent growth in each calendar quarter (or, if the environmental analysis indicates a seasonal market, an objective may be one percent growth in quarter one, one-half percent growth in quarter two, one-half percent growth in quarter three, and two percent growth in quarter four). An issue may be what patrons are charged for the new product or service, compared to the competition.

Marketing Strategies   A strategy is often referred to as a "game plan" to reach goal(s) and objectives. Given the new product or service, such factors as target market characteristics, available funding, and timing should be considered in selecting a strategy. The type of strategy (e.g., product differentiation, mass marketing, niche marketing, or product positioning) and media (e.g., cable, television, print, radio, personal contact, or combination) which will provide the greatest likelihood of success should be selected.

Action Programs   These programs can be viewed as marketing tactics—or how one expects to carry out the strategy. Identify all players and assign each, appropriate responsibility and authority to implement each element of the action program. Answers to the following questions are needed: (a) Who is responsible for each action? (b) What will be done and by whom? (c) When will it be done? and (d) How much will each action cost?

For example, the organization may introduce a new product or service through a month-long multi-media promotion (e.g., tv, radio, newspapers, health care journals). Responsibilities for preparing ad copy, arranging for actors, negotiating prices, proofing print and electronic copy, and coordinating the whole operation should be assigned with clear performance expectations.

Schedules and Controls   Action programs should include schedules which show start and stop dates, when action programs will be evaluated, and the control measures to be used in determining effectiveness. Control measures are tied to the marketing plan's objectives.

Controls are quantifiable measures, such as the actual number of new patrons or telephone inquiries. Controls provide data which answer the question, "How are we progressing right now versus how we projected we would be doing today?" Controls should be valid (they measure what is desired), reliable (over time, measurements are consistent), easy to use, and easy to interpret.

Closing Comments

A final word about marketing plan implementation. The finest marketing plan (or any plan, for that matter) will be rendered invalid and doomed to failure if the plan cannot be implemented by the organization and its people. A major contributor to successful implementation can be isolated in the Action Program, mentioned above. The Action Program must be integrated so as to capitalize upon organizational strengths and minimize the potential negative impact of organizational weaknesses. Further, the action program should mesh with the realities of the external environment. This optimum combination should help the organization achieve successful implementation. A noted marketing authority, Philip Kotler, stated, "many managers think that 'doing the thing right' [implementation] is as important, or even more important, than 'doing the right thing' [strategy]" (Kotler and Armstrong, 1990, p. 58).

SUMMARY

Implementing any plan is challenging. The more change wrought by a plan's implementation, the greater the challenge. The use of organizational development strategies and the employment of negotiation techniques and effective marketing may and often do ease plan implementation.

Organization development strategies have proven useful in lessening resistance to change. The use of a change agent (internal and external) is a particularly powerful device. The change agent can employ structural and behavioral change interventions.

Central to effective plan implementation is effective negotiating. The key to effective negotiation is learning what motivates other people. Negotiation is really turning a potential confrontation into a win-win situation. Mary Parker Follet calls this "integration."

In some instances it may be necessary to develop a marketing plan. Such a plan includes an executive summary, environmental analysis, and a core marketing plan. The executive summary presents the marketing plan's essential concepts. Within an environmental analysis, a situation analysis, and an assessment of the organization's strengths, weaknesses, opportunities, and threats are conducted. The core marketing plan outlines relevant goals and objectives, marketing strategies, action programs, and schedules and controls.

Appendix 9.A

Description of Selected Organization Development Interventions

STRUCTURAL CHANGE INTERVENTIONS

Job Enrichment

An approach that changes the design of a position to enrich the job and provide improved quality of work, based on the incumbent's improved motivation to do outstanding work. It adds more difficult assignments, gives more authority, and permits the completion of whole tasks rather than simple routine parts of a task.

Decentralization

Moving decision-making down the hierarchy to lower levels in the organizational structure. Authority and responsibility must be delegated to the subordinate, as well.

Matrix Organization Design

An organizational structure that is especially effective in project management or when a unit must be responsible for different functions. The matrix overlays a horizontal reporting relationship on the usual vertical relationship.

Program Evaluation Review Technique (PERT)

A planning process that develops a network of activities and events and is usually used in the management of large projects.

Management by Objective (MBO)

A process of establishing goals and objectives throughout an organization, involving all units and individuals; then planning, managing activities, and evaluating performance to ensure achievement of the goals and objectives.

Sociotechnical Design Theory

A theory that emphasizes a relationship between an organization's social system and the technical systems. Emphasis is on the development of independent working groups.

System 4 Management

A technique for analyzing an organization to determine the level of participative management style. The development of interventions to emphasize the effectiveness of participative decision making is the goal of the process.

BEHAVIORAL CHANGE INTERVENTIONS _____

Transactional Analysis

A technique to help employees understand their ego states and thus improve communication methods between individuals.

Laboratory Training

Also referred to as sensitivity training and T-groups. An intervention of experiential exercises with unstructured groups through which the change agent focuses on sensitivity to one's self and interpersonal relations.

The Managerial Grid

A system-wide six-phased intervention based on various styles of leadership behavior with the goal of an ideal leadership style and an organization that supports it. The intervention is looking for proper balance between concern for people and concern for production.

Team Building

An intervention to help work groups understand the process by which they work within their group and with other groups. The goal is more effective team work.

The Johari Window

A technique for identifying and improving the interpersonal communication between individuals. The focus in developing a knowledge of one's self and others.

REVIEW QUESTIONS

1. The OD intervention which is characterized by "moving decision making to lower levels in the organizational structure" is called:
   a. The Johari Window
   b. Transactional Analysis
   c. Sociotechnical Organizational Design
   d. Decentralization

2. It is well known that change affects organizational members in different ways. All of the following statements are correct EXCEPT:
   a. Current methods lead to predictable results.
   b. Organizational systems are classified into two classifications, structural and behavioral.
   c. The structural system consists of two subclassifications, formal and informal.
   d. A system is an organized arrangement of parts which combine to make up the whole.

3. Implementing a plan involves varying levels of difficulty. Listed below are statements concerning plan implementation. All of the following statements are correct EXCEPT:
   a. Knowledge of various systems operating within an organization is essential to successful plan implementation.

b. Implementing a plan which requires change in formal organizational structure is more difficult than implementing a plan which requires change in behavioral systems.

c. Implementing a plan which requires change in formal organizational structure is less difficult than implementing a plan which requires change in the informal organization.

d. First attempt changes in formal organizational structure.

4. When a change agent or planner attempts to identify and assess factors which hinder plan implementation the person is employing which step of OD?
   a. Recognition of need for change
   b. Development of good rapport
   c. Problem diagnosis
   d. Conducting an intervention

5. When a change agent recommends that a job be enlarged, the agent is employing which step of the OD process?
   a. Recognition of need for change
   b. Development of good rapport
   c. Problem diagnosis
   d. Conducting an intervention

6. A change agent has a number of OD intervention options available. All of the following are examples of structural intervention techniques EXCEPT:
   a. MBO
   b. PERT
   c. Job Enrichment
   d. Team Building

7. All of the following are examples of behavioral change interventions EXCEPT:
   a. Transactional Analysis
   b. The Johari Window
   c. The Managerial Grid
   d. System 4 Management

8. The OD intervention which is characterized by "identifying and improving the interpersonal communication style of employees" is:
   a. The Johari Window
   b. Transactional Analysis
   c. Sociotechnical Organizational Design
   d. Job Enrichment

9. The definition, "the harmonious marriage of difference," refers to:
   a. Compromise
   b. Domination
   c. Integration
   d. Reciprocal relations

10. Negotiation involves two or more differing positions on an issue. Concerns such as mistrusting motives or reputation involve what level of negotiation?
    a. First
    b. Second
    c. Third
    d. Fourth

11. The purpose of effective negotiation is:
    a. Compromise
    b. Acceptable agreement
    c. Domination
    d. Win-lose

12. The phrase, "interaction should be depersonalized and all those involved should direct their attention to the situation," refers to which concept?
    a. Change Agent Role
    b. Law of the Role
    c. Law of Roemer
    d. Law of the Situation

13. Which one of the following sections is NOT routinely presented in marketing plans?
    a. Executive Summary
    b. Environmental Analysis
    c. Core Marketing Plan
    d. Impact Analysis

14. The analysis which is conducted prior to new product service introduction is called?
    a. Situation Analysis
    b. SWOT
    c. Action Program
    d. Marketing Strategy

15. Which one of the following is often referred to as a "game plan?"
    a. Action Program
    b. Marketing Strategy
    c. Schedules & Controls
    d. Situation Analysis

DISCUSSION QUESTIONS

1. Select an organization or organizational unit with which you are familiar and which has experienced some change. Compare the process experienced with that outlined in the Stages of Organization Development presented in this chapter.

2. Define the "Law of the Situation" and how it influences negotiation. Describe some negotiation strategies which can be used in meetings.

SECTION *III*

Management Information Systems

10

Management Information Systems: Introduction

Chapter Objectives:

1. Describe the computer in terms of its parts, types, capabilities, and limitations.
2. Describe the recommended relationship between the computer user and an organization's information services department.
3. Describe commonly applied computer security techniques.

Planning and management have always been difficult tasks, but today it is true more so than ever before. Reasons for present day challenges are conditions such as (a) the changing size of organizations, (b) the amount of information available for planners and managers seems limitless, (c) lower-level managers are now expected to make decisions once reserved for middle management, (d) middle-level managers are expected to make decisions once reserved for upper-level managers, and (e) the amount of time in which a decision must be finalized continues to decrease.

Productivity remains a constant concern across all levels of management, regardless of the business. Managers have long focused on improving efficiency ("doing the job right") as well as effectiveness ("doing the right job"). However, there is a limit to the degree management techniques can improve efficiency and effectiveness. Thus, organizations must continue to explore ways to improve productivity through their external and internal operating relationships.

Planners and managers have always relied on information to perform their tasks, so the subject of information utilization is not new. What is relatively new, is the availability of the electronic digital computer to support those decision making tasks. The computer provides decision making support tools enabling solutions to very complex problems in ways that have never been available previously. The computer-based system that offers this information management capability is known as a Management Information System or MIS.

The purpose of this chapter is to acquaint you with MIS components, structure, and current issues. MIS applications are discussed in Chapter 11.

PROGRAM PLANNING AND COMPUTER LITERACY _____

Management experts consider it mandatory that both experienced and novice managers become and remain computer literate. Forecasters are quick to point out that, in the future, those who fail to become computer literate will be unable to perform managerial tasks very well. It won't be a step backwards, but professional peers will be taking giant steps forward while those not computer literate essentially stand in the same place.

The health care environment in which one must operate today is rapidly changing. The challenges posed by change include: (a) managers at the lower and intermediate levels are expected to make decisions once reserved for the upper echelons of the organization, (b) managers are every-day candidates for "information overload" because the amount of information available today is ten times that of ten years ago, and (c) today's managers are expected to make these decisions in half the time afforded their predecessors! The combination of these factors begs for an automated solution to help resolve the challenge.

A Management Information System (MIS), if designed, implemented, and applied properly, can be a valuable support tool for today's health care manager. Therefore, computer literacy is paramount, not just a "nice-to-have" requirement in today's health management world.

The definition of what it will mean to become and remain "computer literate" in the future has changed somewhat over the past few years. Larry Long (1989, p. 9) has stated that the computer literate person will:

a. "feel comfortable in the use and operation of a computer system;
b. be able to make the computer work through judicious development or use of software;
c. be able to interact with the computer—that is, generate input to the computer and interpret output from the computer;
d. understand how computers are impacting society, now and in the future; [and]
e. be an intelligent consumer of computer-related products and services."

Additionally, as is the case today and will be in the future, information is respected and treated as a valuable resource in any competitive organization—identical to the way organizations view people and money. That is, information has a dollar value associated with it in today's competitive world. Also, remember that "knowledge is power" and the conduit for accessing a large part of that knowledge is the organization's Management Information System.

MIS: A CONCEPTUAL FOUNDATION

The computer-based MIS relies on the electronic digital computer as its foundation. The MIS can provide information on the past, present, and future from inside and outside the organization to support both the decision-making and control functions of management.

There are many definitions of a MIS. One definition of a MIS formulated by the authors is, "a communication system that provides managers with reliable, accurate, and timely information that will allow them to control operations." Stoner and Freeman (1989, p. 656) define MIS as, "a formal method of making available to management the accurate and timely information necessary to facilitate the decision-making process and enable the organization's planning, control, and operational functions to be carried out effectively." Aldag and Stearns (1991, p. 606) have defined MIS as, "an integrated system of information flows designed to enhance decision-making effectiveness. Good management information is accurate, timely, complete, relevant in form and content, and available when needed."

What each of these definitions has in common is that a MIS provides reliable information for effective and efficient decision-making in a timely fashion. Before discussing the MIS per se, it is necessary to discuss the very foundation of any MIS—the computer and the support capabilities the computer can provide.

MIS Foundation: The Computer

Those who suffer from "cyberphobia," which is the unwarranted fear of computers, are not alone. Although technically complex, a computer performs very basic functions, such as addition, subtraction, and logic functions as well as input, storage and output operations. If you are unfamiliar with basic computer terms, purchasing a computer dictionary may prove helpful. Also, you may want to take an introductory computer course from a local college or university.

C-A-M-I-O

These five component parts of any computer system are easily remembered with the acronym, C-A-M-I-O. Here the:

- C - *represents the CONTROL UNIT*: Like an orchestra leader, the control unit does not execute the instructions itself; rather, it directs other parts of the system to do so.
- A - *represents the ARITHMETIC AND LOGIC (or "A & L") unit*: This is the only place where computations or logic operations can be performed.

M - represents the MAIN MEMORY UNIT: This is also known as the primary storage unit, internal storage or memory. This unit temporarily holds all data and instructions for processing. All data must first enter main memory before being processed by the computer and all processing results must be placed in main memory before output can occur. Data are held there temporarily because once programs are exchanged, data in the main memory is replaced by the new data. If power is lost to the computer, everything stored in main memory will be lost.

I - represents the INPUT unit (keyboard, wand, scanner, etc.): Unassembled, discrete facts are referred to as "data," and data are what we input into the computer for processing, i.e., data are what go into the computer.

O - represents the OUTPUT unit: Information is sent here for transformation into a product that has meaning to the user such as the printed page or a video display on the screen. Processed data are referred to as "information" because they are now in meaningful and useful form, i.e., information is what comes out of the computer.

The C (control unit) plus the A (arithmetic and logic unit) plus the M (main memory) form the Central Processing Unit (CPU) which, in a sense, is where all processing occurs.

Computer Attributes

Luedtke and Luedtke (1983, p. 9), have described how a computer functions as, "it stores, retrieves, and manipulates data to perform calculations and to make comparisons." The computer (and thus, the MIS) can provide certain benefits based on its functions. When described in terms of system attributes, such as lightning speed, accuracy, reliability, and economy, the benefits are apparent.

Luedtke and Luedtke (1983, pp. 9–16) listed several attributes of the computer which are:

a. *"The computer is fast."* It performs its functions in nanoseconds (one billionth of a second) or picoseconds (one trillionth of a second) and does it so accurately that the unknowing mistakenly attach an element of mystery to the computer. If you held a lighted cigarette in the palm of your hand for a millisecond—a thousandth of a second—you would probably receive a first degree burn; if you held the cigarette for a picosecond, you wouldn't be aware that the cigarette was there!

b. *"The computer stores masses of data economically."* One 3–1/2 inch disk may hold as much information as 400 sheets of paper. Moreover, mass data storage devices provide extraordinary systems capabilities unheard of just a few years ago.

c. *"The computer does repetitive tasks."* Once information and instructions are stored in a computer, it can use them repeatedly for a multitude of applications. This will free the manager to perform other responsibilities.

d. *"The computer is accurate."* Most computer errors are caused by the computer being supplied with the wrong information or the wrong instructions as a result of human error. (Remember the acronym GIGO—garbage in, garbage out— although many misinterpret GIGO to mean: garbage in, gospel out!)

e. *"The computer is reliable."* Although there is some "downtime" for computers, they operate an average of 99.9 percent of the time.

f. *"The system is only as fast as its slowest part."* The INPUT portion of the system remains the slowest component. This is why supermarkets use laser scanners to read prices and why department stores rely on optical wands—all trying to speed up the input part of the system (and also to reduce "human error" in the input process). In the near future, there will be natural language, or voice input capabilities, where the manager just speaks to the computer and it will respond to instructions! In the fall of 1990, a British firm demonstrated such a system with an input dictionary of over 20,000 words.

g. *"The storage capacity is not infinite."* Although the computer can store millions of characters of information, it is limited in disk capacity and main memory capacity although technology has made this less of a concern today. (It's quite easy and inexpensive to increase a computer's memory capability.)

h. *"The computer repeats [or executes] only what it stores."* The computer can process only the data and instructions that have been keyed in or stored electronically.

i. *"The computer doesn't think—yet."* The system cannot make value judgments or be subjective. For example, the computer cannot respond to a query that asks: "Describe the cloudly blue sky." Nor do the computer's vision capabilities replicate those of a human, as users think of human vision capabilities. The computer "visually" compares one object to another, and if a visual match does not exist, it rejects the compared object.

j. *"The computer does only what it's told."* If the instructions are not stored or programmed, the computer cannot execute that command. Regardless of what some cyberphobics think, computer operations are not based on "smoke and mirrors." The computer runs on a series of instructions (called a program) written by a human.

k. *"The computer sometimes has 'bugs'."* No system is error free and it sometimes breaks down (although, 99.9 percent uptime is the standard). Most errors in the system are generated by human error. Computers, like other machines, have scheduled maintenance times to prevent unscheduled downtime and/or to upgrade the system.

l. *"Attitudes create many limitations."* If the managers in charge are willing to encourage experimentation and to tolerate a few errors and/or delays that may result, the system will most likely provide more than just the most elementary benefits. Proficiency (which leads to increased productivity) is a factor of quality training, hands-on experience, and individual initiative as well as some mistakes.

Types of Computers

Computers are sized to fit every need and pocketbook. Computers are generally placed into four size categories for ease of discussion. Today, the distinction among categories and which computer actually fits into which category is very difficult because the boundaries between computer categories change constantly. One caution is appropriate here—do not be deceived by associating the physical size of a computer with its computing capability. For example, today there are laptop computers available that weigh less than 5 pounds; however, they have a computing power greater than some of the much larger computers!

Microcomputers   The smallest category of computers is the microcomputer which, in fact, has several sub-categories, such as the workstation, personal computer (PC) or desk top, laptop (fits conveniently on a lap and weighs between four to sixteen pounds), notebook (can fit into a briefcase and weighs less than four pounds), pocket, and palm top. The most familiar is probably the PC. The name "micro" was applied because these computers could easily fit on a desk top. Due to shrinking technology, another microcomputer, called a sub-notebook, which will weigh about two pounds and be less than half the size of today's notebook computers, will soon emerge. Micros are generally single-user oriented. They use a keyboard for data entry and a visual display terminal or a slow speed printer for output. Micros run on a computer chip called a "microprocessor." Although it is limited in physical size, it is not necessarily limited in computing power.

   There seem to be more technological breakthroughs in the micro area than any other. A review of current literature indicates that industry experts predict that, in the next few years, the laptop computer market will become the hottest competitive market for computer manufacturers. This is good news because computing power will continue to increase, and the cost of utilizing that power will decrease. The bad news may be that the day is rapidly approaching when the manager will be expected to carry the micro everywhere twenty-four hours a day, seven days per week!

Minicomputers   "Minis," such as the DEC VAX or the Unisys U 5000/35, are generally regarded as medium sized computers. Most of them fall between microcomputers and mainframes, although some of the larger ones are called "superminis." Minis are usually designed to handle the processing needs of many users. Minicomputers are more expensive than micros and unaffordable for most individuals. Minicomputers can be equipped with most of the capabilities of the larger mainframes. Minis are used to support the concept of distributed processing where, rather than rely on one large mainframe, several minis are placed at separate remote locations for on-site processing and then connected through telecommunication links like telephone lines.

Mainframe computers   Mainframe computers are large systems, such as the IBM 3090 series, and are pretty much the standard for large organizations. They are more powerful than mini or micro computers. Mainframes can provide central-site processing for several hundred on-line terminals which are simultaneously connected directly to the CPU for processing purposes. Mainframe computers are considered to be general purpose computers which are employed to handle either large, complex or high-volume business processing requirements. They contain large storage capacities, have extremely high processing speeds, and perform their instructions in "millions of instructions per second" (MIPS). Mainframes are frequently rented or leased, whereas minis and micros are usually purchased.

Super computers The largest computers are the super computers, such as the Cray 2. These are few in number and usually only affordable for purchase and operation by large organizations, such as the Centers for Disease Control and Prevention or some of the larger academic institutions (a single supercomputer can cost several million dollars). They are used to process the largest and most complex requirements in such areas as science and math. Super computers are the only category of computers that meet these processing needs because they are designed to run four to ten times faster than a mainframe computer.

Computer Applications

The computer is a very powerful tool that, when employed to its fullest potential, can significantly improve individual and organizational efficiency and effectiveness. Over time, the price of computer hardware has fallen, but its computing power has increased. Software programs have become more "user friendly" and versatile.

Software programs have been developed to perform a variety of applications. These applications include database management, wordprocessing, spreadsheet analysis, and statistical packages. For a full discussion of these and other applications, see *Principles of Information Systems* by Stair (1992).

Electronic bulletin boards and information services are common place, inexpensive, and quite useful. The Public Health Practice Program Office and the National Center for Health Promotion and Chronic Disease Control at the Centers for Disease Control and Prevention in Atlanta, Georgia, can provide information of government sponsored health related electronic bulletin boards and databases. Several guides to commercial bulletin boards have been published and are available from your local bookstore. Be sure to thoroughly research any bulletin board or database prior to participating or paying any money for access.

RELEVANT MIS ISSUES

Relationships: Need Identification

The technical operation of the MIS should not be of concern to the non-technical manager. However, there are certain responsibilities related to the MIS (or computer environment) that necessarily belong to the non-technical manager, such as determining operational requirements and the implementation of a security program.

The manager maintains a responsibility to identify, in matter-of-fact terms, the MIS practical requirements for a department or operation. In other words, the manager must be able to explain to the MIS technician what it is the manager wants the MIS to do for the department. (It is, likewise, the technician's responsibility to develop that technical capability. An "It can't be done" answer from the technician should not be readily accepted.)

Relationships: Service Requests

A MIS operational requirement (a need) is usually recorded on a "service request" form and submitted to the Information Services Department (ISD) of a typical organization. Many managers fail to submit such service requests because it is quite common to have a three year backlog! Regardless, submitting all service requests is encouraged as is having a department member track service requests so they don't get lost.

A particular service request may initially be assigned a low priority rating by the technical staff responsible for upgrades or equipment replacement; however, when a service request is combined with others from within the organization, the request may take on more operational significance. The combining of service requests may be carried out by the MIS technicians or by a users group that meets on a frequent basis to discuss, among other agenda items, upgrades to the MIS.

Tracking service requests are important because the expected life cycle (from "birth to death") for a computer system today is about seven years. As the MIS ages, there will be more and more "patches" applied to the system which will ultimately render it cumbersome and inefficient and in need of replacement. Before replacement, however, the technicians must make some determination about upgrade priorities for the system "patches."

Service request submissions may individually, when coupled with other service requests, result in the immediate identification of a critical "patch" that might otherwise be unrecognized. Also, a clear identification of total system requirements (existing and anticipated) from all departments can signal the need for a new system—a signal which might otherwise remain obscure to top management.

Computer Security: Introduction

Most organizations implement what is known as a "multi-level security program" that addresses both physical security and logical security concerns. Because information is recognized as a valuable resource, security precautions are designed to protect the computer system and data from deliberate or accidental damage (flood, fire, sabotage) or access by unauthorized persons ("hackers").

As the name implies, a multi-level program employs several overlapping layers of security to provide a redundant security capability—a methodology endorsed by security experts.

The first layer of the physical security system frequently uses a bar code reader for the employee's ID at the entrance door, the second layer could be closed circuit television cameras monitoring the building, and a third layer could be the cipher locks on selected entry doors to secure computer operations.

Logical security protection methods include security background checks on employees, assignment of individual employee passwords for access to the computer system, and limited access to information in the computer system.

Despite all these precautions, security breaches occur daily. The more intense computer crimes, such as database intrusion by "hackers" or the planting of computer viruses, are normally the work of computer experts. The biggest threat to a computer facility is its own employees. Most computer crimes are internal, with a large number conducted by Information Service personnel (Long, 1989, p. 399).

Computer Security: Managerial Action

A manager alone is not expected (nor can be) to solve the computer crime problem. However, there are actions that must be implemented to demonstrate commitment to controlling computer crimes in the work environment. Above all, understand and implement the organization's security program. However, if no such program exists or the existing program is ineffective, actions should be taken to establish such a program within a manager's area of responsibility.

Clearly articulate the specifics about the security program to all subordinates. For example, address computer piracy. Piracy is when company owned or licensed programs are copied for personal use. (This is sometimes a "gray" area because many organizations expect their employees to perform official company work at home on the employee's personal computer. To assist in this policy, employees are allowed to copy software for upload onto their personal computers.) If this practice exists in an organization, at a minimum, the manager should explain the implications of unauthorized use of such software.

Clearly state the policy on the use of company computer resources for personal employee use, and, if allowed, when so. (Can the employee type personal letters during the lunch hour, or only before/after the work day, or not at all?) Be certain to state whether or not company policy allows employees to upload their personal software onto company computing resources. (There are computer "games" available that can be exited quickly with one key stroke whenever the boss appears!)

Also, consider unannounced audits of the programs that exist on the computers in a department. Such audits will probably require some assistance from the Information Services Department to ensure that the department's computing resources are authorized. The technicians can also ensure that hardware is not damaged or programs contaminated during the audit.

Security experts also encourage the application of WARNING labels on the outside of each computer video monitor where the labels will be in constant view. The labels serve as a constant visual reminder that computer security is a responsibility of every employee—not just the boss.

Some time should be spent each day walking around the manager's physical area of responsibility. Observe what the "normal" activities are in that work environment and, when something other than "normal" is seen, get involved.

One of the best measures against computer crime is an active "file backup" policy that makes periodic "backup" of all files (copying to another disk or tape) a mandatory event. Most operational personnel shy away from "backup" activities because creating "backup" files represents unproductive time. Consult with computer technicians about establishing a "backup" policy and the best way to implement the policy. Many application programs (e.g., major word processing programs), have built-in backup features that can be activated during the setup phase of program installation. On the larger mini or mainframe computers, backup responsibility should be deferred to the Information Systems Department.

Constantly review and update the computer security program. Laws governing computer and information processing are few, and those that do exist are subject to a variety of interpretations. However, there have been recent court cases in which the copyright owners of major productivity improvement applications, such as wordprocessing software, have won lawsuits involving software piracy within organizations.

Although the legal aspects of computer crime are unclear, prudent behavior suggests that managers are accountable for all operations within their area of responsibility, including computer applications. Lastly, accept as fact that all computing resources cannot be monitored all the time. If a security breach or computer crime does occur, the only legal defense available may be a demonstrable commitment to enforcing established security standards.

Thinking about Buying a Personal Computer?

This has to be one of the most frustrating decisions facing a non-technical user today. There are so many choices available and, unfortunately, there is no single solution to solve the problem. There are considerations, though, when thinking about the purchase of a PC.

When considering the purchase of a computer or an upgrade from an older to a current system, adopt a "needs first" approach. That is, first identify what the user's needs are, needs for both right now as well as for the future. Then and only then, explore what systems are available to meet those needs. Compare several different systems because a purchase normally means about a seven to ten year relationship with the vendor.

One recommended method to learn about the benefits and limitations associated with each system is to compare the equipment of several different vendors. Vendors are willing to explain the benefits of their system—and the limitations of their competitors' systems.

The acronym S-U-P-E-R offers some help in deciding what system to purchase:

S - Be sure the *size* of the system will accommodate your needs now and in the future.

U - Is the system *user friendly*? That is, is the system easy to use with a minimum amount of training?

P - Is it *powerful* enough to meet the needs of your customers? (Yes, computers have different power capabilities.)

E - Is it *expandable* so you can meet future needs?

R - Is it *reliable* so operating time will have a positive, not dysfunctional, effect in meeting your needs?

Remember, before buying a computer or an entire system, first clearly specify what tasks need to be done. Second, research and select the software needed to accomplish those tasks. Finally, research and select the necessary hardware to "run" the selected software.

It is probably not a good idea to rely on a vendor to explain what is needed. If the needed expertise is lacking, consider employing a consultant.

SUMMARY

Managers and planners must be computer literate to function in today's health care environment. The basis of modern management information systems is the computer which comes in a variety of capabilities and limitations. The trend is towards smaller, more powerful computers. As computer based management information systems proliferate, the need to develop strong, effective working relationships with the organization's information services department increases. Managers must take steps to enhance the management information system's security.

REVIEW QUESTIONS

Directions. Read each question very carefully before selecting your answer. There is one correct answer for each question.

1. All of the following are influences which are driving the automation of management information systems EXCEPT:
   a. The size of organizations

    b. The very large amount of information which is available to managers

    c. Lower-level managers make decisions once reserved for senior management.

    d. Middle-level managers make decisions once reserved for senior management.

2. The definition, " a communication system that provides managers with reliable, accurate, and timely information that will allow them to control operations," refers to which term:

    a. Evaluation   c. Management information system

    b. Planning   d. Data recording and reporting system

3. The computer is composed of five component parts. The component which is known as the primary storage unit is the:

    a. Control unit   c. Arithmetic and logic unit

    b. Main memory unit   d. Output unit

4. The component part of a computer which is known for its ability to transform electronic impulses into a product which is understood by the user is the:

    a. Main memory unit   c. Output unit

    b. Arithmetic and logic unit   d. Control unit

5. The type of computer which is the standard for very large organizations is the:

    a. Microcomputer   c. Mainframe computer

    b. Minicomputer   d. Supercomputer

6. The type of computer which is classified as a "notebook" belongs to which one of the following categories?

    a. Minicomputer   c. Supercomputer

    b. Mainframe computer   d. Microcomputer

7. All of the following are considered computer capabilities EXCEPT:

    a. Fast processing speed

    b. Economical cost of data storage

    c. Does repetitive tasks

    d. Does only what is told to process

8. All of the following are considered computer limitations EXCEPT:

    a. Sometimes has "bugs"

    b. Attitudes

    c. Executions are based on stored information

    d. Uneconomical cost of data storage

9. The acronym "CIO" refers to:

    a. Chief Intelligence Officer

    b. Competitor Intelligence Officer

    c. Chief Information Officer

    d. Computer Investment Officer

10. The expected life span of a MIS is about:

    a. Six years   c. Eight years

    b. Seven years   d. Ten years

11. MIS operational needs are expressed in:

    a. Need identification form   c. Service request form

    b. Need request form   d. Service identification form

12. The computer security system which is described as "several overlapping layers of security" is called:

    a. Overlapping system   c. Anti-hacker system

    b. Multi-level system   d. Multi-layer system

13. The biggest source of threat to a MIS is from:

    a. Hackers   c. Customers

    b. Competitors   d. Employees

14. Concerning managerial action respecting MIS security, all of the following statements are accurate EXCEPT:

    a. Use announced audits of software

    b. Use warning labels

    c. Walk around and observe "normal" activity

    d. Adopt a formal "back-up" policy

DISCUSSION QUESTIONS

1. Define what it means to be computer literate. Are you computer literate?

2. Compare and contrast the various types of computers. Which one do you think best meets your current needs and those you anticipate three years into the future? Why?

11

Management Information Systems: Applications

Chapter Objectives:

1. Describe four MIS applications.
2. Describe the relationship between MIS and health planning.

There are ample opportunities to apply MIS capabilities in a work environment—but where? Experts suggest that an environmental analysis can provide answers to this question. Don't be defeated by the term "analysis" because it can be something as simple as personal observation or a more in-depth method, such as the "Critical Success Factors" (CSF) method (Freund, 1988, pp. 20–23).

To focus on opportune MIS applications, step back from the minute-to-minute, day-to-day activities in the work setting and identify those functions which are repetitive in nature (e.g., once an hour, per week, each quarter) and those that are deemed unproductive relative to the skills associated with the health care professional.

For example, in a health care setting, creating work schedules or ordering supplies is repetitive (and laborious), yet unproductive, if a critical care nurse is required to do this instead of providing care. The issue is not whether the "unproductive" activity is needed, but the valuable time required to complete particular tasks at the expense of the direct application of skilled nursing services.

AN ENVIRONMENTAL SCANNING METHOD

The Critical Success Factors (CSF) method requires more analysis than casual observation techniques, but it too can be performed by almost anyone who understands the work environment and who can divide that environment into identifiable activities or components. The CSF method identifies those activities that are critical to achieving the overall goals and objectives within a particular manager's scope of responsibility. (You can relate the critical aspect to a severed carotid artery on a human—better take care of the carotid or all other actions may be in vain!)

To apply the CSF method, assign relative weights of 1 through 10 to work activities. Those activities that are the most *critical* to the successful completion of the work should, for example, be weighted as a 10, 9 or 8 (the carotid deserves a 10!); those with less impact, yet still some significance, would be rated in the range of a 6, 5, or 4; those with little impact would rate a 3, 2, or 1.

For example, the financial transactions of almost any organization are critical to successful operations, thus rating a 10. Another example in a health care setting would be the monitoring of a patient's status, including historical information, that will become part of the patient's medical history. This is probably a 10, whereas using the MIS to set work schedules may be a 5, or the routine ordering of supplies may be a 2. Whatever the weighted values happen to be, the manager can use the analytical information to establish priorities and, hopefully, to improve the productivity of the staff.

In summary, MIS applications should be applied to the critical operations of your department. MIS applications should also focus on those activities that are repetitive in nature and, more than likely, unproductive in terms of accomplishing what it is that the department or unit is supposed to accomplish, i.e., the delivery of health care services.

TRADITIONAL MIS APPLICATION

Traditional management information system produces predefined (i.e., standardized) reports which are used for program monitoring and/or evaluation. These MIS reports are produced by powerful computers or are compiled manually. The tables and figures presented in Chapters 5, 6, and 7 may be seen as examples of reports produced by a traditional MIS. Traditional management information systems will continue to be widely used in health care organizations.

With advances in computer technology and increased experience on the part of users, management information systems have evolved into four other applications, each of which gives planners and managers increased ability to effectively and efficiently utilize the full potential of management information systems.

THE DECISION SUPPORT SYSTEM (DSS)

MIS has been viewed as providing a limited, generic support capability designed to support a specific application such as accounting, inventory control, or human resources management. The MIS, by design, is oriented to support structured problems. Structured problems are those routine problems for which the correct answer is known once the problem has been defined, such as who should be granted credit upon receipt of an application.

It was during the late 1960s when commercial users first began to call for management information systems that could field questions as they occurred to managers, that is, a support tool to handle semi-structured or unstructured problems. A semistructured problem is one for which a partial answer is known; the unstructured problem is one that has not occurred before and for which there is no known ready solution to the problem. In response to this need, the computer industry developed the Decision support system (DSS). Unlike the traditional MIS, a DSS is a set of flexible decision support programs that can be adapted to any decision environment.

Decision support systems facilitate decision making by providing tools for ad hoc data manipulation and reporting. A DSS is similar to an MIS except that the traditional MIS often provides fixed, preformatted information in a standardized way. Unlike the traditional MIS, a DSS always (a) employs interactive terminals (it asks a question and the user responds, etc.), (b) permits posing new questions at a terminal while the user is on-line (connected to the large host computer that contains a database repository of information), and (c) produces irregular reports. Also, a DSS provides programs to be retrieved, processed, and reported in many different ways. Another difference between the DSS and MIS has to do with scope. Most decision support systems are less ambitious in scope (an intentional design feature) than management information systems because DSS designers concentrate on smaller problems rather than developing large, interdependent systems to meet an organization's information needs.

Please recognize that in recent years, the term decision support system has become a computer industry buzzword, a slogan for software vendors touting individual software products. If anticipating the purchase of a DSS, research well before a purchase is made.

The DSS is only successful through the combined effort of man and machine, which is another way of applying the term "semi-structured." By no means does the system solve a problem or replace the health care manager—the human element. The computer is actually a decision *support* system that assists managers in improving their decision making effectiveness. In other words, the system presents suggestions to a manager and then the manager makes the final choice. The human element of working through the decision-making process remains the essential ingredient in the process.

The following five characteristics are typically found in a full-scale decision support system (DSS):

a. The DSS is fully integrated, and able to obtain information from a variety of sources (the marketing department, the finance department, etc.);

b. Analysis is available on a while-you-wait basis (Because one often needs to make short-term, immediate decisions based on the information at hand, most DSS's are used largely to answer questions needed on a given day or week rather than to produce a scheduled weekly or monthly report.);

c. The DSS can produce "What if . . .?" type models—that is, a variety of real-world scenarios or possibilities—to see which outcome the user likes best (This is particularly critical when you must deal with the unexpected. For example, a pharmaceutical products company [as in the Tylenol case] will need to consider the impact of the damage on future sales, the readiness of competitors to take advantage of the situation, and so on. A DSS can support "what-if" questions with a number of simulation models that offer various outcome possibilities.);

d. The DSS crosses departmental functional lines—admissions, accounting, support services and so on—both across the width of the organization and upward and downward within the hierarchy of the organization (Information, analysis, and models from each area are all coordinated for your immediate use.); and

e. The DSS is—that well-worn, overused term—"user friendly" (The user of a DSS is usually a manager, head nurse, facility administrator, or someone at the executive level of the organization—not a data processing guru.).

Such a marvelous DSS system is not cheap. To produce a full-scale DSS, an organization will have to (a) institute sophisticated database management systems; (b) have strong display and graphics capabilities that allow the expression of decision possibilities in visual form, such as charts and graphs; and (c) have modeling tools incorporated in the system, such as risk analysis and forecasting programs. However, experience shows that the benefits from DSS utilization usually far exceed the costs. Currently, an organization may be experiencing huge opportunity costs (lost new business potential) because its MIS is not as versatile as necessary to be able to identify and exploit opportunities. The DSS can provide both contingency and routine decision making capabilities not available from any other source and, thereby, reduce opportunity cost losses. Also, demands from customers for such health care decision support may mandate the application of a DSS!

In practice, particularly to the unknowing or the doubter, the distinction between the MIS and DSS is not always clear. Many see the two terms and capabilities as interchangeable. Also, because the decision-making support capabilities of a MIS and DSS are sometimes incorporated into routine data processing systems, people are justifiably confused about what to call the overall system. Just remember, as previously discussed, a DSS provides much more than just information.

To summarize this discussion, the DSS is a fully integrated package designed to serve a health care manager's needs, which include reviewing the past (reports), examining the present (query) and questioning the future (simulation). In today's health care setting, a mere written report or limited analysis to support current decision-making needs are usually insufficient. With a DSS, a variety of situations (past, present and future) can be analyzed with the same support tool. In essence, the manager is now able to make decisions with a greater degree of expertise than before by using the several decision tools found in the DSS "tool box." Lastly, and to be repetitive, even though DSS offers a number of assistance tools, it is essential to again stress that *by no means should the computer be allowed to make any decision.*

THE EXPERT SYSTEM_____

McLeod (1990, p. 411) distinguishes the expert system from the DSS in two major ways: "First, a DSS consists of routines that reflect how the manager believes a problem should be solved. The decisions produced by the DSS, therefore, reflect the manager's style and capabilities. An expert system, on the other hand, offers the opportunity to make decisions that exceed the manager's capabilities." An expert system is much more complex than the DSS; in fact, it incorporates elements of the most advanced, specialized computer field called artificial intelligence (AI).

According to Long (1989, p. 69), "an expert system is an interactive [it asks you questions and you answer, etc.] 'knowledge-based system' that responds to questions, asks for clarification, makes recommendations, and generally aids in the decision-making process." Long further explains, "expert systems simulate the human thought process. To varying degrees, they can reason, draw inferences, and make judgments" (1989, p. 70). Expert systems have become commonplace today in medical diagnosis. A practical application is in cancer detection or estimating whether or not an individual is prone to suffer from cancer.

Here's how the expert system works: The expert system is created through the cooperative efforts of an AI engineer and one or more experts in a particular area (such as cancer detection), called "domain experts." The AI engineer, who is trained in interviewing techniques, interviews the domain expert(s) and translates everything the domain expert knows into a computer program. The domain expert's knowledge is translated "into factual knowledge and rules to create a knowledge base" (Long, 1989, p. 74). There are additional components of the expert system, but let it suffice for our purposes to say that this expert system is then made available on personal computers for interactive application by a user, such as a cancer specialist attempting to diagnose whether or not a rare cancer is present within a patient. The program will ask questions of the user and, based on the answer provided, will ask additional questions, and so forth until a diagnosis is possible.

A unique capability of an expert system is its ability to "forward-chain" to find a probable result (to reason from the symptoms) or "backward-chain" if the result is known (to reason from the problem back to the cause) (Long, 1989, p. 76). If the symptoms (the "means") are known, the result (the "ends") can be predicted OR if the result is known, the system determines probable causes.

Larry Long (1989, pp. 70–71) identified several benefits that accrue from the use of expert systems which are:

a. "An expert system enables the knowledge of domain experts to be canned [for later use]" (This knowledge can then be distributed for successful use by many non-experts.);

b. "A single expert system can expand the decision-making capabilities of many people" (The decision process can progress more rapidly to the most acceptable solution.);

c. "An expert system can improve the productivity and performance of decision makers" (The solutions to problems will be more consistent because the system itself is consistent.);

d. "An expert system can provide stability and consistency to a particular area of decision-making" (Unlike humans, an expert system responds with exactly the same information to each decision situation.);

e. "An expert system reduces dependency on critical personnel" (This system can contain the thinking from many domain experts so as to benefit others, now and into the future.); and

f. "An expert system is an excellent training tool" (It provides quality training as to how a decision is made within the context of a particular environment.).

Some predict that the expert system is the wave of the future because each user will have an "expert" available to assist in decision-making. However, much work remains to be done in this area in order to expand expert system applications and to bring the cost of such systems within reach of a larger audience.

INTERORGANIZATIONAL DATA EXCHANGE SYSTEMS

One opportunity to improve inter-company (between separate companies) efficiency and effectiveness is through the use of computer-to-computer communications as opposed to less productive methods such as telephone, fax, or older manual systems. The earliest application of computer-to-computer communications methods, known as electronic data interchange (EDI), first appeared in the 1960s. Once the EDI experience base has been established, organizations progress to more advanced applications known as interorganizational systems (IOS) applications.

The following discussion will initially address EDI applications because they can provide leverage to an organization's competitive advantage, and then follow with an introduction to the interorganizational systems capabilities which are available today.

Electronic Data Interchange (EDI)

EDI applications continue to grow among the larger and more profitable Fortune 500 companies in the United States. Moreover, EDI applications are becoming more popular with medium and small organizations because EDI is now an affordable and valuable resource that can immediately improve productivity. Many of these companies achieve a competitive advantage through EDI. Ken Primozic states in his book, *Strategic Choices*, that "the intent of EDI systems is to eliminate time delays, save on people cost, and streamline the administrative process. The management focus on systems that use EDI is to reduce cost and save money" (Primozic, Primozic, and Leben, 1991, p. 84).

EDI is an example of inter-company computing (between separate companies) that links companies, electronically, to better facilitate their required operational interactions. That is, electronic transactions are shipped computer-to-computer using communications facilities. For example, electronic images of actual requisition forms and the subsequent signatures are communicated and documented electronically.

The primary application of EDI systems is in manufacturing, transportation, delivery of products and services, inventory, and accounts receivable. Money is saved through more productive administrative operations.

In an EDI environment, the customer-supplier relationship remains on a transaction-to-transaction basis. There is no structural change in the business relationship between purchaser and supplier.

However, industry experience with EDI documents that as companies expand their applications of electronic data interchange, changes do occur in the business relationship between purchaser and supplier. Purchasers benefit from EDI due "to lower administrative and acquisition costs and reduced inventories." Suppliers benefit by "lower administrative and inventory costs, enhanced cash flow, and help in differentiating products to achieve a competitive advantage" (Primozic, Primozic, and Leben, 1991, pp. 133–134).

In sum, electronic data interchange applications allow organizations to concentrate productivity improvement efforts in administrative support functions to save money, increase efficiency, and enhance organizational flexibility.

Interorganizational Systems (IOS)

The next step with advanced applications of EDI is referred to as interorganizational systems (IOS) because they do change the nature of organizations. IOS lengthens the organization's pipeline into its supplier's organization, which was first created by EDI exchanges.

IOS, in comparison to EDI, extends the purchaser's control into the operation of its suppliers and provides the ability to cause major structural changes to occur in the purchaser/supplier relationship "because such automated systems eliminate many traditional business functions" (Primozic, Primozic, and Leben, 1991, p. 134).

A known IOS application was when a Fortune 500 company provided a notice on January 1st to its suppliers that as of the upcoming September 1st, only those suppliers that utilized IOS capabilities for supply transactions would continue to do business with them.

Here's how IOS works in this resupply example: The purchasing organization sends orders to a supplier's computer. The supplier's computer then sends a shipping notification back to the purchasing company's computer. When the order arrives at the loading dock, a worker verifies that the contents agree with the shipper's bill and causes the purchasing company's computer to transfer monies to the supplier.

This IOS application resulted in a substantial savings in money and time. The supplier no longer needed a worker to record orders because the supplier's computer automatically receives orders. The purchaser has no need for an accounts payable department because orders are paid for when received. The supplier has no need for a conventional accounts receivable function since the funds are electronically transferred as soon as the order is accepted (Primozic, Primozic, and Leben, 1991, p. 134).

Furthermore, this IOS capability is a prerequisite to establishing a just-in-time (JIT) inventory system for the purchaser. A JIT is an inventory control system where inventories arrive just as they are needed. When a threshold is reached, the purchaser's computer automatically orders the necessary materials. A JIT is associated with reduced inventory costs, loss, and theft. These savings, achieved through IOS application, enable many companies to maintain a competitive advantage through increased flexibility and better financial management.

Because IOS applications cause a degree of integration between purchasers and suppliers, an environment is fostered where joint efforts in product development, product quality improvement and other joint ventures may take place.

Interorganizational system applications, when compared to electronic data interchange applications, allow the organization to concentrate on developing "new revenue streams" ('to make money and remain in business') and develop a degree of interdependence, rather than just streamlining existing administrative operations (Primozic, Primozic, and Leben, 1991, p. 136).

LOCAL AREA NETWORKS (LAN)

Intra-company (within the same company) capabilities should exist, most likely via a local area network (LAN). Long states, "a LAN or local net, is a system of hardware, software, and communications channels that connects devices on the same premises [such as a health care center]" (Long, 1989, p. 234). A LAN "permits movement of data, including text, voice, and graphic images, between computers" (1989, p. 234).

A typical LAN supports productivity enhancement efforts through capabilities such as electronic mail, image processing (facsimile and image processing), voice processing (voice message switching and teleconferencing), and office information systems (calendars, conference scheduling, a company directory, and tickler files).

LAN technology continues to improve with an associated reduction in the purchase price and installation of LAN networks. For example, during the fall of 1990, one Japanese firm announced that it would soon market the first PC without any external wires or cables. Imagine the ease of hardware movement and the reduction in associated moving costs made possible with this equipment. There are numerous commercial off-the-shelf LAN networks available today that satisfy the LAN needs of most organizations—and they are affordable.

An intra-company application would be appropriate if an operation or department requires extensive paperwork coordination within the organization (e.g., patient accounting interfaces with admissions, nursing, pharmacy, laboratory, and radiology). Electronic communications will facilitate communications because all paperwork (documents, receipts, historical reports, etc.) can be transferred electronically with great speed and precision.

Potential EDI (and subsequently, IOS) applications, via a LAN, in a healthcare setting include billing insurance companies, storing patient records, electronic mail, and managing accounts receivable or payable. This, in turn, will improve productivity by allowing professional staff members to devote their time to the delivery of quality, skilled patient care (or support functions) rather than "doing paperwork."

MANAGERIAL PLANNING WITH AN MIS

Management analysis indicates that those in the upper echelons of an organization spend over half of their time in the planning function. Operations oriented managers are spending increasing time and effort in planning. When the appropriate applications are implemented within your organization, a management information system can be of assistance in planning and managing efforts.

When compared to earlier management information systems, a modern MIS can have an impact on the quality of plans by:

a. *Causing faster awareness of problems and opportunities*: An MIS can quickly signal out-of-control conditions requiring corrective action when actual performance deviates from what was originally planned. New plans can then be implemented to correct the situation(s). Masses of current and historical internal and external data can be analyzed by use of statistical methods to detect opportunities. Data stored on-line may permit one to probe and query a database and to receive quick replies to planning questions.

b. *Enabling the devotion of more time to planning*: Use of an MIS can reduce the need to wade through mounds of routine reports. More time and attention can be devoted to analytical and logistical matters associated with planning.

c. *Permitting the timely consideration to more complex relationships between and among decision alternatives* An MIS gives the ability to evaluate more possible alternatives. The manager will then be able to consider more of the internal and external variables that may have a bearing on the outcome of these alternatives. Also the planner may do a better job of identifying and assessing the probable economic and social affects of different courses of action. The awareness of such affects, of course, influences the ultimate decision. In the past, the manager or planner had to make oversimplified assumptions if resulting decisions were to be timely. Now consideration and examination of more complex relationships are possible. These relationships are increasingly being highlighted through the use of charts, maps, and other visual presentations displayed on screens of graphic terminals. In short, an MIS can furnish a manager or planner with planning information that could not have been produced at all a few years ago or that could not have been produced in time to be of any value.

d. *Assisting in decision implementation*: When a decision is made, an MIS can assist in the development of plans that will be needed to implement the decisions which have been made. Computer-based techniques to schedule project activities have been developed and are now widely used. Through use of such techniques, health care resources can be utilized and controlled more effectively.

When planning (or managing) any health program, consult with the organization's chief information officer. That individual should be able to suggest additional ways the organization's MIS may be of assistance. Given today's available technology and the reasonable dollar cost to attain that technology, there is no real justification to continue manual management information systems or to maintain massive amounts of paper files or transaction records. Nor is it acceptable not to have the information needed to plan and manage effectively.

SUMMARY

There are five widely used management information system applications in the health care environment. The applications are the traditional application, the decision support system, the expert system, the interorganizational data exchange systems, and the local area network. As these applications continue to mature and as others evolve, the effect on managerial planning will be profound. To remain efficient and effective, the planning manager must become and remain familiar with a variety of management information system applications.

REVIEW AND APPLICATION QUESTIONS

Directions. Read each question very carefully before selecting your answer. There is one correct answer for each question.

1. The type of management information system application which incorporates "AI" is:

    a. Traditional MIS   c. DSS
    b. Computer networks   d. Expert systems

2. The type of management information systems which produces standardized reports which are routinely used in program monitoring is:
    a. LAN   c. Expert systems
    b. Traditional MIS   d. DSS

3. The type of management information system which is based mostly on personal computers is:
    a. Computer networks   c. Expert systems
    b. DSS   d. Traditional MIS

4. The environment in which you work is fairly stable and the challenges you confront are predictable. Which one of the following types of MIS are you most likely to be using?
    a. DSS   c. Computer networks
    b. Traditional MIS   d. Expert systems

5. The Critical Success Factors method is used in:
    a. DSS   c. Environmental Scanning
    b. IOS   d. Traditional MIS

6. Concerning the application of MIS, each of the following statements is considered correct EXCEPT:
    a. Applied to critical operations of the department
    b. Applied to repetitive tasks
    c. Applied to less critical departmental operations
    d. Applied to supplement managerial decision-making

7. The MIS application designed to address semi-structured problems is:
    a. IOS   c. Expert system
    b. DSS   d. LAN

8. Computer-to-computer interface between companies, such as a purchaser and supplier, is known as?
    a. EDI   c. LAN
    b. IOS   d. DSS

9. The MIS application most likely to be used in medical diagnosis is:
    a. EDI   c. DSS
    b. IOS   d. Expert system

10. Concerning EDI benefits, each of the following statements is true EXCEPT:
    a. Purchaser benefits include lower administrative and acquisition costs.
    b. Suppliers benefit from enhanced cash flow and inventory costs.

    c. Changes in the business relationship do not occur.

    d. For suppliers, customer product needs are differentiated.

11. Which of the following MIS applications is the oldest?

    a. Traditional MIS   c. Expert system

    b. DSS   d. IOS

12. Concerning differences between DSS and Expert systems, each of the following statements is accurate EXCEPT:

    a. DSS consists of routines that reflect how the manager believes a problem should be solved.

    b. Expert systems offer the opportunity to make decisions that exceed a manager's capabilities.

    c. A DSS is more complex than an Expert system.

    d. An Expert system is an interactive, knowledge based system.

13. Concerning IOS, each of the following statements is accurate EXCEPT:

    a. Changes the nature of organizations

    b. Extends the purchaser's control into the supplier's operations

    c. Accounts receivable and/or payable functions remain unaffected

    d. Are more advanced than EDI

14. Concerning potential impact of MIS applications to planning, each of the following statements is accurate EXCEPT:

    a. Causing faster awareness of problems and opportunities

    b. Increases time available for planning

    c. Evaluates decision alternatives more thoroughly

    d. No real impact on decision implementation

Case 1: Northwest Health Center Operations Report

Read the following health services utilization report and answer the following questions.

    The Northwest Health Center operates several services during the second shift as it is located in a large urban city. Presented below are two Level 1 reports from the Center's management information system concerning the Center's primary care clinic. Level 1 reports are prepared for operations level health services managers.

    Listed under each column number are the following: (1) service provided, (2) actual number of services provided, (3) ratio of number of services provided to position, (4) the desired service delivery performance standard per position, and (5) the percentage over (positive) or under (negative) the actual number of provided services (or duration in minutes for questions 18–20) are, as compared to the desired performance standard. Maintaining performance standards is considered essential to ensuring quality patient care.

Report Level: 1 (Operations Manager)
Service: Primary Care Clinic
Subject: Service/RN Staffing Ratios for Second Shift

(1) Service	(2) # Provided	(3) Actual Service/Position	(4) Performance Standard	(5) % +, −
Intake	120	40:1	30:1	+33
Prep	120	23:1	25:1	−9
Nur. Assess	80	20:1	10:1	+100
Exit Inter.	90	30:1	25:1	+20

15. Does the second shift appear to be short-staffed?
    a. No
    b. Yes
    c. Insufficient information provided
    d. Don't know

16. Which service is experiencing the *largest* demand relative to desired staffing?
    a. Intake
    b. Patient prep
    c. Nursing assessment
    d. Exit interview

17. Which service is experiencing the *least* demand relative to desired staffing?
    a. Intake
    b. Patient prep
    c. Nursing assessment
    d. Exit interview

Report Level: 1 (Operations Manager)
Service: Primary Care Clinic
Subject: Service Duration in Minutes for Second Shift

(1) Service	(2) # Provided	(3) Actual Service/Duration	(4) Performance Standard	(5) % +, −
Intake	NA	11	15	−27
Prep	NA	10	11	−9
Nur. Assess	NA	13	15	−13
Exit Inter.	NA	10	13	−33

18. Which service appears to be the *most* hurried?
    a. Intake
    b. Patient prep
    c. Nursing assessment
    d. Exit interview

19. Which service appears to be the *least* hurried?
    a. Intake
    b. Patient prep
    c. Nursing assessment
    d. Exit interview

20. If you were the operations manager for the primary care clinic, what would you do given these data? (Essay)

DISCUSSION QUESTIONS

1. How does a decision support system (DSS) differ from a traditional management information (MIS)? How might you use a DSS in planning a health program?

2. How might an expert system be used in planning health programs?

3. How might you use any of the applications presented in this chapter to improve productivity where you work or have worked?

4. How do management information systems influence health program planning? Can you think of other influences?

SECTION *IV*

Sample Operations Level
Health Plans

Case I

Title: Navalley Hospital Biomedical Equipment Repair Program

Submitted By: Douglas E. Thomas
               Health Services Equipment Manager
               Supply Division

Budget Requested: $70,208.65

Submission Date: 19 November 1991.

This case was contributed by Ensign Douglas Thomas, USN. The name of the institution and individuals in this case were changed. There is no intention that this plan refers to any health services organization existing any where or at any time.

I. PROJECT DESCRIPTION

Statement of the Problem

In this 200 bed facility, there are approximately 1,000 pieces of medical equipment that could break down and disrupt daily activities. Because the nearest medical equipment repairman is located approximately 600 miles away from this facility, equipment failures often go unattended for extended periods. In the event vital, lifesaving equipment becomes unusable, the repairman must attempt to assess the problem over the phone, then schedule a trip to conduct necessary repairs, all the while hoping a correct diagnosis was made based solely on the description given. The end risk is that at some point someone who could have been saved will be in danger of death because a piece of equipment needed by the medical staff was inoperable due to poor maintenance or other preventable reasons.

Project Justification

All equipment repairs and routine maintenance must await scheduled quarterly visits by a qualified repair technician. To have an onboard, qualified repairman would increase efficiency, obviate the need for multiple back-up systems, minimize risk to patients and staff by having properly functioning equipment, and increase life expectancy of costly equipment through proper maintenance. Our current level of equipment in inventory is approximately $2.5 million. Overall, expenditures for replacement and repairs of this equipment could be reduced by roughly 33 percent with an active preventive maintenance and repair program (Hampton, 1991).

Summary of Project Methodology

An equipment repairman and an assistant will be hired to locate, identify, inventory, repair, and maintain all important pieces of medical equipment. The repairman will also be responsible for concentrating on priority, lifesaving equipment to ensure proper functioning or replacement at all times. Additionally, the repairman will train a select group of staff members in fundamental maintenance techniques. The repair team will also develop a computer data-base equipment inventory and maintenance tracking system designed to provide an automatic listing of equipment with their respective scheduled maintenance dates.

Summary of Expected Outcomes

An increase in efficient use of costly equipment will be achieved. More importantly, critical, lifesaving equipment will be regularly monitored to ensure operational functioning and availability at all times. The proposed training program will give staff members the requisite knowledge needed in basic preventive maintenance. This will allow users to better appreciate the needs of the equipment and, consequently, treat the equipment with more care. The final outcome of this program will provide a system where routine maintenance schedules and an equipment inventory system are readily available on a data-base system for easy tracking.

Evaluation Element

Appendix I, Sub-Appendix A is the program's evaluation grid; this identifies each objective and activity with their respective indicators of attainment and methodology of documentation. To ensure program efficiency, quarterly status reports, on all aspects of the repair teams' responsibilities, will be provided to the Health Services Equipment Manager (HSEM), who will also have a first hand working knowledge of the organization's equipment status. These data will be collected by interviewing department supervisors and staff maintenance trainees to determine overall efficacy of the program. Other methods of collection will be direct observation, equipment inspection, and conversations with pertinent personnel.

The Biomedical Equipment Repair Technician (BMERT) will be responsible for ensuring that operational plans are developed and implemented. The BMERT will develop a data-base system (with the aid of the HSEM and other "experts") designed to track equipment inventory and scheduled preventive maintenance or replacement dates.

The HSEM will be responsible for maintaining a high level of responsiveness from the repair team. The HSEM will also be responsible for ensuring that adequate progress within the proposed project is achieved. In concert with these responsibilities, all gathered information will be compared with data collected at earlier phases in the project and analyzed on a statistical and practical basis to determine developing trends on a quarterly basis. Reports, which keep management apprised of results, will be generated through an integrated management information system (MIS) and will detail areas such as response time when assistance is needed, equipment down time, extended life of traditionally short-lived equipment, and reduced needs for major repairs. A Gantt Chart, attached as Appendix I, Sub-Appendix B, also has been developed to aid in program tracking and management.

II. PROGRAM BUDGET

Navalley Hospital biomedical equipment repair program budget

Personnel-Positions		$43,000.00
Biomedical Repair Technician	$26,000.00	
Repair Assistant	17,000.00	
Personnel-Fringe Benefits		12,654.00
Biomedical Repair Technician	$ 7,681.50	
Repair Assistant	4,972.50	
Office Support		11,714.65
Office Equipment	$ 6,031.11	
Office Furniture	4,820.61	
Office Supplies	361.99	
Telephone	500.94	
Educational Materials		590.00
Instructional Equipment	$ 40.00	
Printed Materials	500.00	
Other	50.00	
Continuing Education		2,000.00
Other Costs		250.00
Contingency Fund	$ 250.00	
	Total =	$70,208.65

BUDGET JUSTIFICATION STATEMENT _____

Personnel Positions

Biomedical Equipment Repair Technician (BMERT) and Assistant BMERT are estimated to cost $26,000 and $17,000 respectively (Hopke, 1991, p. 14). This level of
compensation is needed to attract and retain technicians capable of accomplishing the
following: (1) maintain and repair existing equipment; (2) properly and expediently
install newly acquired equipment; and (3) evaluate potential equipment for reliability,
functionality and cost-effectiveness. The Repair Assistant is to assist the repairman and
ensure a smooth operating department. The task proposed cannot be effectively
accomplished with only one technician. Position descriptions are in Appendix I,
Sub-Appendix C.

Personnel-Fringe Benefits

Personnel-Fringe benefits are needed to attract and retain high quality technicians and
will cost $12,654. This figure was reached by multiplying annual salaries times
Navalley's fringe benefit rate of 29.43 percent.

Office Support

Current office space is available and no additional funds will be needed for this. Specialty
equipment, tools, and work shop furniture will cost approximately $11,714.65. This
figure includes a computer and printer that will be needed to manage the data-base
program. All items are needed to conduct on-site repairs in an efficient and cost effective
manner and allow for adequate information processing (Nazario, 1991).

Educational Materials

Flip charts, quick reference guides, and instructional video tapes are required in training
employees and are estimated to cost $590.00 (Nazario, 1991).

Continuing Education

Continuing education is required to maintain repair skills in concert with the development of new equipment, repair techniques, and tools used, thus allowing the BMERT to
provide repairs on state-of-the-art equipment. This is estimated to cost $1,000 for each

BMERT, for a total of $2,000. Because seminars for repairmen are typically out of the local area and normally last three to four days, costs include round trip air fare, hotels, and meals (Nazario, 1991).

Other Costs

Contingency fund is estimated at $250 and is needed to offset items that may unexpectedly need replacing (e.g., a tool that breaks), or non-routine purchases of local supplies (e.g., wire, nuts, bolts, etc.).

Appendix I

Sub-Appendix A

PROGRAM EVALUATION GRID

Program Goal: To develop a system which eliminates, or reduces to a minimum, medical equipment failures and down time, and establish a functioning preventive maintenance program between 1 January 1992 and 1 March 1993.

Program Objectives	Attainment Indicator	Method of Gathering Data
1) To have a qualified medical repair technician and assistant selected and hired by 1 March 92.	Repairman and assistant hired.	Statement by Personnel department
a) Determine necessary qualifications, skills, and competitive pay level of qualified repairman by 15 Jan 92.	Statement of attainment	Copy of data from Personnel department
b) Place ads in national and regional newspapers and trade journals by 21 Jan 92.	Copy of ads	Collect copies of newspapers and journals
c) Contact regional job placement centers inquiring about possible candidates by 21 Jan 92.	Statement of attainment	Report of results

Program Objectives	Attainment Indicator	Method of Gathering Data
d) Select and hire candidates by 1 Mar 92.	Signed employee contract	Copy of contract
2) To have 100% of "lifesaving equipment on line and/or checked out for maintenance requirements by 1 May 92, and all other necessary equipment scheduled for repairs by 1 Sep 92.	Statement of attainment	Copy of report
a) Identify all lifesaving equipment by 5 Mar 92.	List of equipment	Copy of list
b) Locate and inspect each piece of equipment by 15 March 92.	List with location and status of equipment	Copy of list
c) Determine which pieces of equipment need repair/ maintenance, and set priorities/schedules by 20 Mar 92.	List of equipment	Copy of list
d) Order necessary parts and repair critical equipment by 1 May 92.	Invoice of parts ordered	Copy of invoice
e) Repeat process for non vital equipment and have completed by 1 Sep 92.	Statement of attainment	Copy of list and invoice
f) Perform scheduled routine maintenance inspections on all equipment according to required frequency from 1 Apr 92 to 1 Mar 93.	Equipment maintenance history record	Copy of records
3) To have 90% of selected staff members trained in basic maintenance techniques by 1 Mar 93.	List of employees trained	Copy of list
a) Interview department heads and floor supervisors and select capable staff members by 15 May 92.	List of selected employees	Copy of list

Program Objectives	Attainment Indicator	Method of Gathering Data
b) Develop curriculum by 1 June 92.	Curriculum	Copy of curriculum
c) Schedule, advertise, and conduct 10 training sessions from 1 June 92 to 1 Mar 93.	Training schedule and flyers for advertising	Copy of schedule and flyers
d) Conduct follow-up visits to departments with recently trained personnel from 1 June 92 to 1 Mar 93.	Statement of attainment & feedback reports	Copy of feedback
4) To effectively manage the repair/maintenance process on an ongoing basis, but at least quarterly from May 92 to Feb 93.	Statement of attainment	Report on effectiveness of program
a) Inventory 100% of major pieces of equipment by 1 Sep 92.	Inventory list	Copy of inventory
b) Construct data-base inventory and maintenance records system covering 100% of major equipment items by 1 Mar 93.	Functioning data base program with maintenance dates	Demonstration of program
c) Conduct monthly site visits on repair division to ensure continued progress from 1 Mar 92 to 1 Mar 93.	Report detailing findings and date visited	Copy of report
d) Provide quarterly progress reports to Health Services Equipment Manager on an ongoing basis between 31 May 92 and 28 Feb 93.	Statement of attainment	Copy of reports

Appendix I

Sub-Appendix B

PROGRAM MANAGEMENT GANTT CHART _____

	1992 Jan	Feb	Mar	Apr	May	Jun	Jul	Aug	Sep	Oct	Nov	Dec	1993 Jan	Feb	Mar
Objective															
1a	*														
1b		*													
1c		*													
1d			*												
Objective															
2a			*												
2b			*												
2c			*												
2d				*											
2e								*							
2f				*-----											-----*
Objective															
3a					*										
3b						*									
3c						*-----									-----*
3d						*-----									-----*
Objective															
4a									*						
4b														*	
4c				*-----											-----*
4d					*			*			*			*	

Figure I.1   Navalley Hospital Plan Gantt Chart

Appendix I

Sub-Appendix C

POSITION DESCRIPTIONS

Position: Biomedical Equipment Repairman

Education: Minimum high school graduate who has successfully completed formal training in one of the nationally recognized institutions for biomedical repairman.

Experience: At least 10 years experience in complete repair, installation, and evaluation of equipment. Must be computer literature in a data base program.

Duties: Repair and install all biomedical equipment
Develop computerized inventory system
Develop computerized tracking system for preventive maintenance program
Conduct training sessions
Assist in equipment purchase
Evaluate equipment selected for purchase
Manage biomedical repair division
Order supplies and replacement parts
Perform other duties as assigned

Position: Biomedical Equipment Repairman Assistant

Education: Minimum high school graduate with mechanical background in medical field. Preference will be given to formally trained, entry level technician.

Experience: 2 years experience in medical equipment repair or graduate of formal biomedical equipment repair school with no expeience.

Duties: Assist repairman
Perform basic repairs (non-complex)
Maintain and update equipment inventory
Perform basic preventive maintenance
Perform other duties as assigned

REFERENCES _____

Hampton, R. Telephone interview. 10 December 1991.

Hopke, W. (1991). *Encyclopedia of Careers and Vocational Guidance*. Chicago: Ferguson.

Nazario, T. Telephone interview. 23 October 1991.

Case II

Title: West Coast Health Care Systems Cancer Center, Cancer Patient Support Services (CaPSS)

Submitted By: Donna Bryan, RN
                 Nurse Manager, Oncology Unit

Budget Requested: $217,557

Submission Date: 1 June 1991

This case was contributed by Donna J. Bryan, RN, OCN. The name of the institution and individuals in this case were changed. There is no intention that this plan refers to any health services organization existing any where or at any time.

I. PROJECT DESCRIPTION _____

Statement of the Problem

Advances in detection and treatment of cancer have transformed a nearly fatal disease to one that is often curable.[1] There are now over three million individuals in the United States who are five-year cancer survivors.[2] Because people live longer with cancer, a sizeable cancer popuulation within Florida, Long County, and in the West Coast Health Care Systems (WCHS) service area has been established. In 1995, projected new cancer cases in Long County alone is estimated at 6,313. (See Appendix II, Sub-Appendix A.) In 1991, about 1,100,000 people will be diagnosed as having cancer in the United States and an estimated 73,000 people in Florida.[2] (See Appendix II, Sub-Appendix B.)

     Cancer is an emotional disease. Physicians and healthcare professionals who provide services directed at meeting the emotional needs of patients often are more successful than those who concentrate on providing simply the technological services. Many cancer centers in the Smith Bay area have devoted money, time, and energy to developing technologies and clinical services, as well as psychological support services. However, what has more recently been identified is that programs that appeal to the emotional nature of disease entities are sometimes more successful in attracting patient populations than institutions that merely provide technological expertise.[3]

Presently, WCHS offers the following psychosocial support services:

1. Two support groups conducted weekly at the Center for Radiation Therapy.
2. "I Can Cope," an American Cancer Society (ACS) sponsored education program conducted three or four times annually at the Center for Radiation Therapy.
3. Liaison and referral services with Hospice and ACS.
4. Crisis intervention counseling for inpatients and outpatients on a part-time basis.

The above services are currently provided by a part-time oncology counselor employed by the Center for Radiation Therapy.

When comparing the existing resources presently available to those being offered by our competition, it becomes quite clear that WCHS has a very inadequate psychosocial oncology program. The subcommittee on psychosocial oncology noted the following deficiencies:

1. Lack of a centralized, coordinated referral base for physicians or patients resulting in a detriment in the continuity of care.
2. Fragmented services due to a lack of full-time staff attention specifically for oncology resource management.
3. Very little, if any, community support for patients and family facing emotional turmoil of this dreaded disease.
4. No evaluation for inpatients and the lack of individual or family counseling.
5. Other than minimal crisis intervention, professional counseling is unavailable to outpatients.
6. Ongoing staff education and support programs are nonexistent.[4]

Such psychosocial service deficiencies in the WCHS Cancer Center are expected to continue unless program expansion is undertaken.

Project Justification

The proposed Cancer Patient Support Services (CaPSS) will support patients and their families who are coping with cancer by offering individual and group sessions with trained counselors as well as educational programs.[5] CaPSS's philosophy relates to Bernie Siegel's Exceptional Cancer Patient (ECaP) program, which believes that psychosocial services, especially in an oncology program, play an integral role in the healing process of both patient and family.[6] This philosophy was reinforced by several WCHS physicians participating in the Oncology Task Force who believe cancer patients must have access to psychosocial services to assist them and their families to adjust to the disease and its treatment while maintaining an optimal quality of life.[5]

CaPSS program significantly supports the mission of WCHS (to provide superior health care at a reasonable cost) by recognizing the emotional needs of cancer patients and realizing these correlate directly with the physical needs of this patient population. CaPSS will strengthen the multi-disciplinary team in providing superior health care.

Accurate, up-to-date statistics on the number of cancer patients in this demographic area are difficult to obtain. The best estimate is from the 1990 Cancer Facts and Figures information compiled by the ACS. Based on a Long County population number of 850,000:

1. 11,050 persons are estimated to be alive and "cured" from cancer.
2. 11,900 persons are estimated to be under medical care for cancer.
3. 1,700 is the estimated number of persons who will die of cancer.
4. 3,400 is the estimated number of new cancer cases.
5. 1,700 is the estimated number who will be cured from cancer.[4]

In 1989 and 1990, 3,412 new cancer patients were introduced into the WCHS Cancer Center for initial diagnosis and treatment.[7]

At present, there is no other cancer center in Long County offering to the community a psychosocial program such as CaPSS. The potential for increase in market share for quality cancer treatment is beyond limitations. By attracting more cancer patients to WCHS, CaPSS can generate revenue from patients who are unaffiliated and/or those cancer patients seeking to change affiliation to WCHS. Even though most of the CaPSS programs would be offered at a minimal cost, if any, to cancer patients, it is being evaluated on the basis of CaPSS generating revenue through other departments and clinical services, particularly those linked with cancer care (e.g., Radiation, Radiology, Pharmacy, Laboratory). It is reasonable to project a minimum self-referral from non-service geographic locations of one patient per week or fifty-two patients per year. The CaPSS program is designed to make WCHS Cancer Center emotionally preferable to the patient and family. It is projected that by 30 April 1992, WCHS Cancer Center will provide a comprehensive multi-disciplinary support and education program for cancer survivors and families under the CaPSS program.

Proposed Project Methodology

The proposed program will require a total of four full-time equivalent masters-prepared social workers with oncology experience. The current part-time ECaP oriented counselor will assume the full-time position of program coordinator, thereby coordinating all activities involved in acquiring additional oncology counselors. The managers of the Center for Radiation Therapy and the Oncology Inpatient Unit will give final approval for selection of candidates. To address the needs and correct the deficits identified, the coordinator will develop a job description addressing referrals, provision of individual, family and group counseling services, patient education, staff education and support, and resource management. The CaPSS program coordinator will report to the Center for Radiation Therapy manager.

The CaPSS department will develop and implement three additional weekly support groups to cancer patients already affiliated with WCHS and other cancer patients in the service area. The purpose of these support groups may focus on areas such as bereavement and/or women with breast cancer. The upper county service area has been identified as a target for location of support groups. The CaPSS coordinator will supervise all support group activities, identifying the appropriate skilled counselor to lead specific groups. A bi-monthly newsletter will be formulated by the CaPSS department directed to patients and families living with cancer and as an information source about CaPSS program activities.

Professional staff of the proposed program will design; schedule and conduct at least two, three-day workshops directed toward cancer patients and families; and schedule and conduct one specifically directed toward other professionals. The education component would encompass areas related to home care, physical appearance, travel tips for the health impaired, latest state-of-the-art treatment options, exercise, nutrition, humor, and imagery. Outside professionals will be employed to conduct special topic sessions to help attract attendance.

Expected Outcomes

It is expected as a result of the proposed program, WCHS will increase its market share in the treatment of cancer. Six support groups of ten participants weekly or fifty patients per week can potentially generate new patients in the system. Individual and family counseling sessions are projected at 50 per week, or 2,400 per year. Psychosocial services enchance patient care, complement the ability of the oncology physician to treat the total patient, and heighten the quality of the overall cancer program.[5] In addition, the two, three-day workshops with a registration fee of $200 per participant, will generate revenue to offset expense. But most of all, WCHS, with the CaPSS program, will be a forerunner in comprehensively addressing the emotional aspect of living with cancer. It will place WCHS on the cutting edge of in extremely competitive market place.[4]

Evaluation Element

Presented in Appendix II, Sub-Appendix C is the proposed program's evaluation grid, which presents each program objective, service target, and activity along with the indicator(s) which will indicate attainment as well as how data will be obtained.

Generally, records of employment, copies of documents and advertisement materials, and quarterly reports by program staff will be used to evaluate goal, objective, and service target attainment. An impact evaluation (August) will be conducted with reports to the Service Champion. The effectiveness of the program on inpatient care will be evaluated by tracking inpatient length of stay compared to the past two years.

The manager of the Center for Radiation Therapy will be responsible for maintaining the quality of administrative and financial services and practices of the proposed program in accordance with WCHS policy and procedure. The CaPSS coordinators will be responsible for maintaining the quality of counseling, support groups, and educational services in accordance with WCHS standards of practice.

The CaPSS coordinator will be responsible for developing the program's management information system with respect to tracking data related to goal and objective attainment. Data will reside within a database capable of tabulating and reporting data in pre-configured formats. WCHS Data Processing Center will be available to assist in data collection upon request.

The program's management objective requires continuous monitoring and quarterly reporting. The development of the program's management information system ensures objective attainment. A Gantt chart has been developed to facilitate project management. (See Appendix II, Sub-Appendix D.)

Marketing Element

Program services and educational programs will be marketed via CaPSS newsletters, WCHS Foundation publications, newspaper advertisements, and printed brochures. In the 1992 cancer center marketing budget, monies have been allocated for advertisement of cancer program services. WCHS physicians, cancer patients and families, and program staff will inform other cancer patients of program services.

II. BUDGET DESCRIPTION

CaPSS program budget

	Annual Salary Rate	#FTE	Total Annual Salary
1. Personnel			
a) Position Title			
CaPSS Coordinator	$29,806	1.0	$ 29,806
Oncology Counselor II	28,059	3.0	84,177
Medical Secretary	22,339	1.0	22,339
	Total Salary Requested:		$136,322

	Annual Salary Rate		#FTE	Total Annual Salary
Fringe Benefits:			Worker's Compensation & Insurance	
b) Position/Salary	Salary	FICA (7.65%)	(28%)	Total
CaPSS Coordinator	$29,806	$2,280	$ 8,346	$10,626
Oncology Counselor II	$84,177	$6,440	$23,570	$30,010
Medical Secretary	$22,339	$1,709	$ 6,255	$ 7,964
		Total Fringe Benefits Requested:		$48,600

2. Travel:

Position	Mileage	Per Diem Rate	Common Carrier	Meals	Total
Supervisor	$ 50	$ 800	$1,000	$210	$ 2,060
Oncology Counselor II	$100	$1,600	$2,000	$420	$ 4,120
Oncology Counselor I	$ 50	$ 800	$ 500	$105	$ 1,455
			Total Travel Requested:		$ 7,635

3. Office Support:

Office Equipment	$ 4,500
Office Furniture	$ 2,000
Office Supplies	$ 3,500
Total Office Support Requested:	$ 10,000

4. Educational Materials:

Equipment	$ 5,000
Printed Materials	$ 5,000
Total Educational Materials Requested:	$ 10,000

5. Other Costs:

Marketing Expense	$ 5,000
Total Other Costs Requested:	$ 5,000

Summary of Proposed Budget:

Personnel:	$184,922
Travel:	7,635
Office Support:	10,000
Educational Materials:	10,000
Other Costs:	5,000
Total Costs:	$217,557

BUDGET JUSTIFICATION STATEMENT _____

Personnel Positions

Five full-time FTE positions are needed: a CaPSS Coordinator, three Oncology Counselors, and a Medical Secretary. (See Appendix II, Sub-Appendix E for Administrative Flow Chart.) Such a staffing pattern is needed to attain program goal, objectives and service targets. There will be a transfer of the funds for CaPSS Coordinator from the Center for Radiation Therapy to CaPSS program budget since the .5 FTE is currently funded by the Center for Radiation Therapy. Positions are funded for 12 months.

Personnel—Fringe Benefits

Using WCHS's standard fringe benefit rate of 35.65 percent of salary, the cost of program employee fringe benefits is $48,600. Such a fringe benefit package is required to attract and retain high quality personnel.

Travel

Travel is projected to cost $7,635, which includes mileage; per diem, including hotel costs and professional seminar registrations; meals (standard WCHS rates), and travel costs to a national meeting for oncology psychosocial support and one other professional seminar.

Office Support

There are no office space or utility costs charged to the project as there are two offices vacant, one in radiation outpatient center and one on the oncology unit. Office equipment (computer bundle, printer, typewriter, and software) costs are projected to be $4,500. Office furniture costs (computer desk and 6 chairs) are projected to be $2,000. Three executive style desks are available through WCHS warehouse at no extra cost. Office supply costs are projected to be $3,500. Telephone equipment, service, and lines are available to the program at no charge. These materials are needed to support the program.

Educational Materials

The projected costs of audio-visual equipment is $5,000 (two VCRs with monitor and stand, audio cassette tapes for relaxation, cancer support education videos, books relating to psychosocial needs of cancer patients). These tapes and books will be used as support and educational materials for patients, families, and staff. Printed materials (educational workshops, materials, newsletters, fliers, and support group pamphlets) are projected to cost $5,000. The materials are essential to accomplish educational objectives and service targets.

Other Costs

Marketing expense is estimated at a cost of $5,000 (newspaper advertising and professional journal advertising for educational workshop and program awareness).

Appendix II

Sub-Appendix A

Projected new cancer cases in 1995 using county population and incidence rates

	Population	Rate/100,000	New Cases
Long	921,315	685.2	6,313
Pasco	332,625	791.3	2,632
Hernando	125,626	763.1	959
Hillsborough	974,441	386.7	3,768
Total	2,354,007		13,672

Source: State Government, 1991.

Appendix II

Sub-Appendix B

MAGNITUDE OF THE CANCER PROBLEM IN FLORIDA_____

Florida has the highest crude incidence and death rates for cancer of all states, including the District of Columbia and Puerto Rico.

Cancer is the leading cause of death among persons aged 25 to 64.

Florida has the fifth highest mortality in the nation for cervical cancer among black women.

Cancer, while rare in children, is second only to accidents as a leading cause of death from birth to fifteen years of age.

There are about 60,000 new cases of cancer diagnosed in Florida every year.

Children under 15 years of age account for an average of over 300 cases of cancer annually in Florida.

The number of new cases of cancer in Florida increases by about 2,500 each year, or nearly 5 percent.

More than half of all new cancer cases are among Florida's elderly population.

Between 1981–87, there were an average of 9,088 cases diagnosed and 7,849 deaths each year due to lung cancer.

By the year 2000, close to 80,000 cases of cancer will be diagnosed each year in Florida.

Elderly Florida residents will account for 68 percent of all cancers diagnosed in the year 2000.

Less common cancers are becoming more common with the increase in immigration, migration, and overall population of the state.

Source: Cancer in Florida—Seven-Year Overview. Florida Cancer Data System, Florida Department of Health and Rehabilitative Services, p. 3.

Appendix II

Sub-Appendix C
Program Evaluation Grid

Program Goal: To provide a comprehensive multi-disciplinary support and education program for cancer survivors and families by 30 April 1992.

Program Objectives	Attainment Indicator	Method of Data Gathering
1. Increase the number of oncology counselors by three full-time equivalents for inpatient and outpatient services by 21 November 1991.	Employed	Personnel profile copy. Authorization to hire form copy.
a. Develop an oncology counselor job description by 1 October 1991.	Job description	Job description copy
b. Advertise for positions in local newspapers and direct mail fliers to social workers' professional organizations between 1 October 1991 and 31 October 1991.	Newspaper ads Direct mail	Copy of newspaper ads. Organization receives direct mail flyer.

Program Objectives	Attainment Indicator	Method of Data Gathering
c. Interview applicants by program managers and employ selected counselors by 21 November 1991.	Scheduled interviews	Interview schedule and summary of interview.
d. Promote the present oncology counselor to coordinator of program by 1 November 1991.	Statement of Attainment	Copy of promotion statement.
2. Develop and implement three additional support groups for patients and families by 30 January 1992.	Group schedule	Copy of group schedule.
a. Identify the type of support groups defining purpose by 7 December 1991.	Statement of attainment	Copy of defined groups.
b. Schedule meeting locations, dates and times by 10 December 1992.	Statement that activity completed	Copy of schedule, meeting locations and times.
c. Assign counselors to lead individual support groups by 21 December 1991.	Statement of attainment	Copy of coordinator's assignment report.
d. Advertise via a newsletter and brochure the support groups to the public by 20 January 1991.	Statement of attainment	Copy of newsletter and brochure.
3. Develop and conduct three-day workshops for patients, families and other professionals by 30 April 1992.	Number of workshops held	Report of workshop held and participant count.
a. Develop an educational curriculum to educate patients and families on coping strategies with cancer by 28 February 1992.	Curriculum	Copy of curriculum

Program Objectives	Attainment Indicator	Method of Data Gathering
b. Develop an educational curriculum to educate professionals on coping techniques for the cancer survivors by 28 February 1992.	Curriculum	Copy of curriculum
c. Employ other "professionals" to provide topic sessions within the curriculum by 28 February 1992.	Statement of attainment	Copy of agreement statement, work shop schedule, and speakers' list.
d. Schedule, advertise, and conduct two educational three-day workshops between 28 February 1992 and 30 April 1992.	Statement that activity completed. Number of workshops held. Number of attendance.	Copy of advertisement material, and schedule. Report of workshops being held.
4. To effectively and efficiently manage the CaPSS program between 1 October 1991 and 31 July 1992.	Statement of attainment	Report of project attaining objectives on budget.
a. Develop an administrative flow chart of CaPSS program by 21 November 1991.	Flow chart	Copy of flow chart.
b. Develop a patient and family counseling referral policy and procedure by 15 December 1991.	Policy and procedure	Copy of policy and procedure.
c. Report to the Service Champion quarterly between 1 October 1991 and 31 July 1992.	Statement of attainment	Quarterly reports.
d. Report impact evaluation results by 1 August 1992.	Statement of attainment	Copy of report

Appendix II

Sub-Appendix D

PROGRAM MANAGEMENT GANTT CHART _____

Months	1991			1992							
	Oct	Nov	Dec	Jan	Feb	Mar	Apr	May	Jun	Jul	Aug
Objective											
1a	*										
1b	* ---*										
1c			*								
1d		*									
Objective											
2a			*								
2b			*								
2c				*							
2d				*							
Objective											
3a						*					
3b						*					
3c						*					
3d						* ----------*					
Objective											
4a		*									
4b			*								
4c			*			*		*			
4d										*	

Figure II.2   WCCHCS Gantt Chart

Appendix II

Sub-Appendix E
CaPSS Program
Administrative Flow Chart
Manager Center for Radiation Therapy

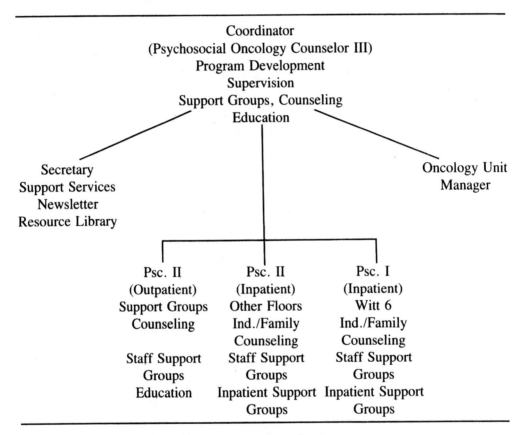

Figure II.2   CaPSS administrative flow chart

REFERENCES

1. Holland, Jimmie C. and Julia H. Rowland, ed. *Handbook of Psychooncology.* New York: Oxford University Press, 1989, p. 101.
2. Cancer Facts and Figures—1991. American Cancer Society, Inc., p. 1.
3. Wilson, Elizabeth, Cashing in on Cancer. Florida Trend, June 1990.

4. WCHS Psychosocial Oncology Subcommittee Report, 1990.
5. Gustafson, Meta H., MA, LMHC. Psychosocial Oncology Counselor, WCHS. Interview.
6. Siegel, Bernie S. Peace, *Love and Healing*. New York: Harper & Row Publishers, 1989
7. Hill, Jane, CTR, Supervisor, WCHS Tumor Registry, Interview.

ANSWERS TO REVIEW AND/OR APPLICATION QUESTIONS

Chapter 1

1. b, 2. d, 3. b, 4. c, 5. a, 6. b, 7. d, 8. d, 9. b, 10. d.

Chapter 2

1. c, 2. d, 3. b, 4. a, 5. c, 6. a, 7. b, 8. d, 9. a, 10. a, 11. b, 12. d, 13. b, 14. b, 15. b, 16. c, 17. d.

Questions 18–23.

18. d. Statement 18 is the most global of all the statements (18–23) and states the organization's reason for existence.
19. c. Statement 19 is less global than statement 18, and does not meet the definition requirements to be an objective.
20. d. Statement 20 meets the definition requirements of an objective, but calls for *600* unknown laboratory tests which is more general than statement 21.
21. c. Statement 21 calls for the processing of *200 pregnancy* tests weekly which is much more specific than statement 20.
22. c. Statement 22 describes the expected output of a single position.
23. a. Statement 23 describes specific action which will be undertaken, but does not meet the definition requirements of an objective nor does it call for specific level of output by a particular position.

Questions 24–30.

24. b. Statement 24 meets the specifications of an objective.
25. b. Statement 25 calls for management of the project.
26. b. Of all of the statements (24–30), 26 is the most general and suggests the organization's reason for existing.
27. c. Statement 27 describes an action which must be done. It states no anticipated service level; nor does it meet the definition requirements of an objective.
28. d. Statement 28 is fairly general but is less so than statement 26. Statement 28 does not meet the definition requirements for an objective.
29. c. Statement 29 states in quantifiable terms what a specific position is supposed to do within a specific time.
30. a. Statement 30 states in quantifiable terms what the program is supposed to do for a specific group by a specific date.

Chapter 3

1. d, 2. d, 3. c, 4. d, 5. b, 6. c, 7. b, 8. c, 9. b, 10. d.

Chapter 5

1. b, 2. c, 3. b, 4. c, 5. a.

CASE 1: NORTHWEST COUNTY HEALTH DEPARTMENT

6. c. Almost 58% of the population is over 45, 75% white, and 17% have incomes over $35,000.
7. a. Almost 58% of the population is over 45 and 64% have a high school diploma or less.
8. d. 71% have income less than $25,000 and there is only a 3% difference between males and females.

CASE 2: HIV RISK CATEGORIES

9. a. Whites, Non-Hispanic account for 54% of US cases and 48% of Florida cases.

10. c. 3253 divided by 191,601 equals 1.697% or 1.70%.

11. c. 21% + 6% equals 27%.

Chapter 6

1. d, 2. c, 3. d, 4. d, 5. b, 6. b, 7. d, 8. b, 9. c.

CASE 1: DIABETES IN XYZ COUNTY

10. b. The prevalence rate for the east side of the county was 217/100,000 compared to the west's 153/100,000.

11. a. The incidence rate for the west side of the county was 57/100,000 compared to the east's 33/100,000.

12. b. The median age cohort for diabetes related mortality among males on the east side was 55–59, while the west's was 60–64.

13. c. The median age cohort for diabetes related mortality among females is the same for both sides of the county.

14. b. The male to female diabetes related mortality in the east was 3 to 1, while the west's was 2 to 1.

CASE 2: HEART DISEASE IN XYZ COUNTY

15. b. The east side of the county has the highest incidence rate.

16. a. The west side of the county experiences later dates of onset and a later mortality median cohort for males. The female mortality median cohort did not differ.

17. b. In the east side of the county, females experience an earlier age of onset (67) than in the west side (71).

18. b. In the east side of the county, males have an earlier median age cohort (60–64) than in the west side (65–69).

19. a. In the west side of the county, the male to female mortality ratio is 2:1 as opposed to the east's 1:1.

Chapter 7

1. d, 2. b, 3. c, 4. c, 5. c, 6. b, 7. a, 8. d, 9. c, 10. b, 11. d, 12. a, 13. c, 14. c, 15. a, 16. d, 17. c.

CASE 1: NORTHWEST COUNTY PUBLIC HEALTH DEPARTMENT_____

18. a. Almost 31% of county residents are on a public (i.e., government) health insurance program with 34% private pay and the average household income for the county is $11,500 with an average household size of 3.6 persons.
19. c. Private physicians provide 43% of the county's health services. Given the information, there is no way of knowing about the potential for doubling public health service delivery. When one considers that 91% have access to automobile transportation, it would appear that residents have geographical access even though 82.5% of providers are located in the county seat. If transportation access were more limited "c" would not be accurate.
20. a. The county is rural. Since average household income is $11,500 and average household size is 3.6 persons, average per capita income is about $3,194.

CASE 2: INPATIENT LOS_____

21. a, 22. b, 23. b, 24. d.

Chapter 8

1. c, 2. d, 3. d, 4. b, 5. c, 6. d, 7. b, 8. c., 9. d, 10. b

Chapter 9

1. d, 2. c, 3. b, 4. c, 5. d, 6. d, 7. d, 8. a, 9. c, 10. a, 11. b, 12. d, 13. d, 14. a, 15. b.

Chapter 10

1. c, 2. c, 3. b, 4. c, 5. c, 6. d, 7. d, 8. d, 9. c, 10. b, 11. c, 12. b, 13. d, 14. a.

Chapter 11

1. d, 2. b, 3. a, 4. b, 5. c, 6. c, 7. b, 8. a, 9. d, 10. c, 11. a, 12. c, 13. c, 14. d.

CASE 1: NORTHWEST HEALTH CENTER _____

15. b. Three of the four services being provided are between 20 and 100 percent over performance standard.
16. c. Nursing assessment is 100% over performance standard.
17. b. Patient prep. is 9% below performance standard.
18. d. The exit interview is 33% below performance standard.
19. b. Intake is 9% below performance standard.
20. Answers probably will vary. Based upon these data, the clinic appears to be short-staffed given available staffing patterns relative to service demand. Staff appear to be rushing through tasks, thus possibly compromising the quality of patient care. Steps taken could include: (a) increasing available staff, (b) reducing service demand, (c) revising the performance standards, or (d) ignoring the situation.

Glossary

ACTIVITY: Action steps which must be executed in order to achieve a specified objective.

ANALYTICAL EPIDEMIOLOGY: "[It is] designed to examine associations, commonly putative or hypothesized causal relationships. [A]n analytic study is usually concerned with identifying or measuring the effects of risk factors, or is concerned with the health effects of specific exposure(s) . . . [and unlike] descriptive [epidemiology], does not test hypotheses" (Last 1988, pp. 5–6).

ARITHMETIC SCALE LINE GRAPH: "One where an equal distance represents an equal quantity anywhere on the [y] axis, but not necessarily between the axes [x and y]" (Ferrara, 1980, p. 94).

BUDGET JUSTIFICATION STATEMENT: A statement, keyed to each line-item, which briefly explains the rationale for it.

CAUSE SPECIFIC RATES: Those with reference to a specific disease or condition, e.g., AIDS death rate per 100,000 population.

CASE SPECIFIC RATES: Those with reference to a specific epidemiological investigation, e.g., AIDS case fatality rate between 1987 and 1991 in Miami.

CHART: "A method of presenting statistical information symbolically using only one coordinate" (Ferrara 1980, p. 102) The most commonly employed chart is the bar chart.

CLOSED QUANTITATIVE INTERVIEWS: "Questions and responses are determined in advance. Responses are fixed; respondent chooses from among these fixed responses" (Patton, 1980, p. 206).

CLUSTER OR AREA SAMPLING: A type of stratified sampling where the stratification is in clusters. Cluster sampling is usually reserved for large studies. Cluster sampling is subject to the possibility of significant error, as it really is a sample of samples.

CRUDE RATES: Reflect morbidity and/or mortality without reference to a specific disease, condition, or set of cases, e.g., crude death rate per 100,000 population.

CONVENIENCE SAMPLING: A convenience sample is composed of those subjects who are most convenient.

DECISION SUPPORT SYSTEM: A set of flexible decision support programs that can be adapted to any decision environment.

DESCRIPTIVE EPIDEMIOLOGY: "[The] study of the amount of and distribution of disease within a population by person, place, and time" (Mausner and Bahn, 1974, p. 43).

DIMENSIONAL SAMPLING: In dimensional sampling, all the variables of interest (e.g., gender, race, age category, and HIV status) are specified. In the sample, at least one subject with each characteristic, and every possible combination, must be present.

ELECTRONIC DATA INTERCHANGE (EDI): An MIS application of inter-company computing (between separate companies) that links companies, electronically, to better facilitate their required operational interactions. That is, electronic transactions are shipped computer-to-computer using communications facilities.

EPIDEMIOLOGY: "The study of the distribution and determinants of health-related states or events in specified populations, and the application of this study to the control of health problems" (Last 1988, p. 42).

EVALUATION RESEARCH: "A method of evaluating a process to enable judgments to be more accurate and objective" (Rubinson and Neutens 1987, p. 12).

EXPERIMENTAL EPIDEMIOLOGY: "Equated with randomized control trials" (Last 1988, p. 45)

EXPERT SYSTEM: An MIS application which "offers the opportunity to make decisions that exceed a manager's capabilities" (McLeod 1990, p. 411).

GANTT CHART: A management device that helps a planner and/or program manager to efficiently and effectively manage program operations.

GOAL: "A long-range specified state of accomplishment toward which programs are directed" (Reinke 1988, pp. 66–67).

GRAPHING: "A method of showing quantitative data using a coordinate system (for our purposes, usually x and y)" (Ferrara 1980, p. 92).

HEALTH SERVICES RESEARCH: The application of social science research principles and methods to the study of health services organization, distribution, delivery, utilization, management, and finance.

HISTOGRAM: "A graph used only for presenting frequency distribution of quantitative data. There is no space between the cells . . . on a histogram" (Ferrara 1980, p. 96).

IMPLEMENTATION EVALUATION: Within implementation evaluation, the program's implementation experience is investigated, documented, and analyzed.

IMPACT EVALUATION: Within impact (summative) evaluation, both the intended and unintended final effect(s) of the program are researched, recorded and analyzed.

INCIDENCE: "A measurement of only the new cases of a disease or other event during a given period" (Austin and Werner, 1974, p. 61).

INFORMAL CONVERSATIONAL INTERVIEW: "Questions emerge from the immediate context are asked in the natural course of things; there is no predetermination of question topics or wording" (Patton, 1980, p. 206).

INTEGRATION: "The harmonious marriage of difference" (Fox and Urwick, 1982, p. xxv). Refers to conflict resolution. Integration means invention of new solutions and the realization that neither party must give up a portion or all of what they want.

INTERORGANIZATIONAL SYSTEMS (IOS): Lengthens the organization's pipeline into its supplier's organization, which was first created by EDI exchanges.

INTERVIEW GUIDE APPROACH: "Topics and issues to be covered are specified in advance. In outline form, interviewer decides sequence and working of questions in the course of the interview" (Patton, 1980, p. 206).

LAW OF THE SITUATION: Meaning that interaction should be depersonalized and all those involved should direct their attention to the situation (Fox and Urwick, 1982, p. 29).

LOCAL AREA NETWORK (LAN): "Is a system of hardware, software, and communications channels that connects devices on the same premises [such as a health care center]" (Long, 1989, p. 234).

LINE-ITEM BUDGET: A budget which organizes projected expenditures by line item category. It is the simplest and most common form of budgeting used in operations planning.

MANAGEMENT INFORMATION SYSTEM (MIS):   A communication system that provides managers with reliable, accurate, and timely information that will allow them to control operations.

MAINFRAME COMPUTERS: Mainframe computers are large systems and standard for large organizations. They are more powerful than "Mini" or "Micro" computers. Mainframes can provide central-site processing for several hundred on-line terminals which are simultaneously connected directly to the CPU for processing purposes.

MEAN: The average of a numerical distribution.

MEASURES OF CENTRAL TENDENCY: Refers to the mean, median, and mode within a distribution.

MEDIAN: The category or actual score above which 50% of the cases fall and below which 50% of the cases fall.

MICROCOMPUTERS: The smallest category of computers which has several sub-categories such as the workstation, personal computer (PC) or desk top, laptop (fits conveniently on a lap and weighs between 8–16 pounds), notebook (can fit into a briefcase and weighs less than 8 pounds), pocket, and palm top. The PC is probably the most familiar. The name "Micro" was applied because these computers could easily fit on a desk top.

MINICOMPUTERS: Usually designed to handle the processing needs of many users. Minicomputers are more expensive than micros and unaffordable for most individuals. Minicomputers can be equipped with most of the capabilities of the larger mainframes.

MISSION: "The purpose of an organization" (Robbins, 1991, p. 220).

MODE: The value that occurs the most frequently in a numerical distribution.

NONPROBABILITY SAMPLING: "The probability that a person will be chosen is not known, with the result that a claim for representativeness of the population cannot be made" (Rubinson and Neutens, 1987, p. 90).

OBJECTIVE: "Stated in terms of achieving a measured amount of progress toward a goal, specifies:

> **WHAT:** The nature of the situation or condition to be attained.
> **HOW MUCH:** The quantity or amount of the situation or condition to be attained
> **WHEN:** the time at or by which the desired situation or condition is intended to exist.
> **WHO:** the particular group of people or portion of the environment in which attainment is desired, and
> **WHERE:** the geographic area to be included in the program" (Reinke 1988, pp. 66–67).

OPERATIONS PLANS: "Plans that specify how overall objectives [i.e., goals] are to be achieved" (Robbins 1991, p. 194).

ORGANIZATION DEVELOPMENT: "Systematic process to change the culture, systems and behavior of an organization, in order to improve the organization's effectiveness in solving its problems and achieving its objectives" (Rush, 1974, p. 32).

PERFORMANCE STANDARDS: Essential in operations health planning as they determine what is the acceptable level of productivity each worker is to render.

PERIOD PREVALENCE RATE: Measures prevalence during a specified period of time, e.g., an entire month (Ferrara, 1980, p. 137).

POINT PREVALENCE RATE: Measures prevalence at a given instant in time, e.g., a single day (Ferrara, 1980, p. 137).

POPULATION: A specifically defined universe of persons, skills, objects, or other things to be studied.

PREVALENCE RATE: "A measurement of all cases of disease or other events prevailing at a given time. It includes new cases and old cases" (Austin and Werner, 1974, p. 62).

PROBABILITY SAMPLING: "Those wherein the probability of selection [into a sample] of each respondent, or address, or even object, is known" (Rubinson and Neutens, 1987, p. 85).

PROCESS EVALUATION: Within process (formative) evaluation, the program's progress is examined, documented, and analyzed. Process evaluation is conducted from the time program is implemented to its termination.

PROGRAM BUDGET: Costs are distributed, along line-items, across specific programs.

PURPOSIVE SAMPLING: The researcher selects those subjects who best meet the purpose of the study. This strategy does not rely on random selection (i.e., probability) but on the experience and judgment of the researcher.

QUOTA SAMPLING: This strategy is equivalent to stratified random sampling, except that subjects are not randomly selected. Once the quota of sample subjects is set for each strata, the researcher finds eligible subjects to fill each quota.

RANDOM SAMPLING: This is the simplest form of probability sampling. Subjects are selected without bias or prior exclusion. Every subject has an equal chance of being included in the sample.

RATIO: "Used to express the relationship of one number to another" (Austin and Werner, 1974, p. 62).

SAMPLE: A specifically defined subset of a population which is selected through various means.

SERVICE TARGET: Specified level of service volume directed towards a defined target population.

SNOWBALL SAMPLING: In this sampling strategy, subjects possessing the desired characteristics are interviewed. These subjects suggest others possessing the same characteristics, who are in turn interviewed. This process continues until the desired sample size has been reached.

STANDARDIZED OPEN-ENDED INTERVIEW: "The exact wording and sequence of questions are determined in advance. All interviewees are asked the same basic questions in the same order" (Patton, 1980, p. 206).

STRATEGIC MANAGEMENT: "The process by which top management determines the long-run direction and performance of the organization by ensuring that careful formulation, proper implementation, and continuous evaluation of the strategy takes place" Holland (1989, p. 3).

STRATIFIED RANDOM SAMPLING: "The population is broken down into nonoverlapping groups called strata, and then a simple random sample is extracted from each stratum" (Rubinson and Neutens, 1987 p. 86).

SUPER COMPUTERS: The largest of computers. These are few in number and usually only affordable for purchase and operation by very large organizations.

SYSTEMATIC SAMPLING: "The selection of specific items in a series according to some predetermined sequence. The origin of the sequence must be controlled by chance [random]" (Rubinson and Neutens, 1987, p. 86).

REFERENCES

Abramson, J. H. (1988). *Making sense of data: A self-instruction manual of the interpretation of epidemiological data.* New York: Oxford University Press.

Aday, L. A. & Shortell, S. M. (1988). "Indicators and predictors of health services utilization." In Stephen J. Williams and Paul R. Torrens (Eds.) *Introduction to Health Services* (3rd ed.) (pp. 65–72). Albany, NY: Delmar.

Aldag, R. J. & Stearns, T. M. (1991). *Management* (2nd ed.) Cincinnati: South-Western Publishing Company.

Anderson, S. B., Ball, S., & Murphy, R. T., (1981). *Encyclopedia of educational evaluation.* San Francisco: Jossey-Bass Publishers.

Austin, D. F. & Werner, S. B. (1974). *Epidemiology for the health sciences.* Springfield, IL: Charles C. Thomas.

Babbie, E. R. (1990). *Survey research methods* (2nd ed.). Belmont, CA: Wadsworth Publishing Company, Inc.

Berk, M., Cunningham, P., & Beauregard, K. (1991). "The health care of poor persons living in wealthy areas." *Social Science Medicine, 32* (10), 1097–1103.

Bogdan, R. C. & Biklen, S. K. (1982). *Qualitative research for education: An introduction to theory and methods.* Boston: Allyn and Bacon, Inc.

Campbell, D. T. & Stanley, J. C. (1963). *Experimental and quasi-experimental designs for research.* Chicago: Rand McNally College Publishing Company.

Cohen, W. A. (1991). *The practice of marketing management* (2nd ed.). New York: MacMillan Publishing Company.

Cornelius, L., Beauregard, K., & Cohen, J. (1991). *Usual sources of medical care and their characteristics* (AHCPR Pub. No 91-0042, National Medical Expenditure Survey Research Findings 11). Rockville, MD: Agency for Health Care Policy and Research, US Public Health Service.

DeFriese, G. H., Ricketts, T. C., & Stein, J. S. (1989). *Methodological advances in health services research.* Ann Arbor, MI: Health Administration Press.

DeLozier, J. E. & Gagnon, R. O. (1991). *National ambulatory medical care survey: 1989 summary* (Advance Data from Vital and Health Statistics, no 203). Hyattsville, MD: National Center for Health Statistics.

Denver, G. E. (1991). *Community health analysis* (2nd ed). Gaithersburg, MD: Aspen Publishers.

Dilman, D. A. (1978). *Mail and telephone surveys: The total design method.* New York: Wiley-Interscience.

Ferrara, C. (1980). *Vital and health statistics: Techniques for community health analysis* (DHHS Publication No. 1980-640-185/4455). Washington, DC: US Government Printing Office.

Fisher, R. & Ury, W. (1983). *Getting to yes: Negotiating agreement without giving in.* New York: Penguin Books.

Fox, E. M. & Urwick, L. (1982). *Dynamic administration: The collected papers of Mary Parker Follett.* New York: Hippocrene Books, Inc.

Freund, Y. P. (1988). "Critical success factors." *Planning Review,* July/August 1988, 20–23.

Frey, J. H. (1983). *Survey research by telephone.* Beverly Hills, CA: Sage Publications.

Graves, E. J. (1991). *1989 summary: National hospital discharge survey* (Advance Data from Vital and Health Statistics, no 199). Hyattsville, MD: National Center for Health Statistics.

Gibson, J. L., Ivancevich, J. M., & Donnelly, J. M. (1988). *Organization: Behavior, structure, process.* Plano, TX: Business Publications, Inc.

Harvey, D. F. & Brown, D. R. (1992). *An experimental approach to organization development.* Englewood Cliffs, NJ: Prentice-Hall, Inc.

Henderson, M. M. & MacStravic, R. E. (1982). "The growing role of epidemiology in health services. In Anne Crichton and Duncan Newhauser (Eds.) *The New Epidemiology—A Challenge to Health Administration* (pp. 15–30). Arlington, VA: Association of University Programs in Health Administration.

Henerson, M. E., Morris, L. L., & Fitz-Gibbon, C. T. (1987). *How to measure attitudes.* Beverly Hills, CA: Sage Publications.

Irizarry, A., (1988). "Utilization of health services among the Puerto Rican elderly: gender considerations." *Puerto Rican Health Science Journal, 7,* 215–224.

Isaac, S. & Michael, W. B. (1981). *Handbook in research and evaluation.* San Diego: Edits Publishers.

Kosecoff J. & Fink, A. (1982). *Evaluation basics: A practitioner's manual.* Beverly Hills, CA: Sage Publications.

Kotler, P. & Armstrong, G. (1990). *Marketing* (2nd ed). Englewood Cliffs, NJ: Prentice-Hall, Inc.

Last, J. M. (1988). *A dictionary of epidemiology* (2nd ed.). New York: Oxford University Press.

Lavrakas, P. J. (1987). *Telephone survey methods: Sampling, selection, and supervision*. Beverly Hills, CA: Sage Publications.

Lilienfeld, A. M. & Lilienfeld, D. A. (1980). *Foundations of epidemiology*. New York: Oxford University Press.

Long, L. (1989). *Management information systems*. Englewood Cliffs, NJ: Prentice Hall

Luedtke P. & Luedtke, R. (1983). *Your first business computer*. Bedford, MA: Digital Press.

Mausner, J. S. & Bahn, A. K. (1974). *Epidemiology: An introductory text*. Philadelphia: W. B. Saunders Co.

McLeod, R. (1990). *Management information systems* (4th ed.) Chicago: Science Research Associates, Inc.

McMillan, J. H. & Schumacher, S. (1984). *Research in education*. Boston: Little Brown and Company.

National Center for Health Statistics (1990). *Health United States, 1990 and prevention profile*. Hyattsville, MD: Author.

Nelson, C. (1991). *Office visits by adolescents*. (Advance Data from Vital and Health Statistics, no 196). Hyattsville, MD: National Center for Health Statistics.

Patton, M. Q. (1980). *Qualitative evaluation methods*. Beverly Hills, CA: Sage Publications.

Patton, M. Q. (1990). *Utilization focused evaluation* (2nd ed.). Beverly Hills, CA: Sage Publications.

Pelfrey, S. H. (1992). *Basic accounting and budgeting for hospitals*. Albany, NY: Delmar Publishers.

Primozic, K. Primozic, E. & Leben, J. (1991). *Strategic choices*. New York: McGraw-Hill.

Reinke, W. A. (1988). *Health planning for effective management*. New York: Oxford University Press.

Remington, P. L., Smith, M. Y., Williamson, D. F., Anda, R. F., Gentry, E. M. & Hogelin, G. C. (1988). "Design, characteristics, and usefulness of state-based behavioral risk factor surveillance: 1981–1987." *Public Health Reports, 103* (4), 366–375.

Ries, P. (1991). *Characteristics of persons with and without health care coverage: United States, 1989*. (Advance Data from Vital and Health Statistics, no 201). Hyattsville, MD: National Center for Health Statistics.

Ries, P. & Brown, S. (1991). *Disability and health: Characteristics of persons by limitation of activity and assessed health status, United States, 1984–88*. (Advance Data from Vital and Health Statistics, no 197). Hyattsville, MD: National Center for Health Statistics.

Robbins, S. P. (1990). *Organization theory: Structure, design, and applications* (3rd ed.) Englewood Cliffs, NJ: Prentice Hall.

Robbins, S. P. (1991). *Management* (3rd ed.) Englewood Cliffs, NJ: Prentice Hall.

Robey, D. & Altman, S. (1982). *Organization development.* New York: Mac-Millan.

Rubinson, L. & Neutens, J. J. (1987). *Research techniques for the health sciences.* New York: MacMillan.

Rue, L. W. & Holland, P. G. (1989) *Strategic management: Concepts and experiences* (2nd ed.). New York: McGraw-Hill.

Rush, H. M. F. (1974). "Organization development: A reconnaissance." In Gordon L. Lippitt, Peter Longseth, & Jack Mossop (Eds.), *Implementing organizational change* (p. 27). San Francisco: Jossey-Bass.

Schulz, R. & Johnson, A. C. (1990). *Management of hospitals and health services.* St. Louis: C. V. Mosby Company.

Shillinglaw, G. & Meyer, P. E. (1983). *Accounting: A management approach* (7th ed.). Homewood, IL: Richard D. Irwin, Inc.

Stair, R. M. (1992). *Principles of information systems.* Boston: Boyd and Fraser Publishing Company.

Stoner, J. A. F. & Freeman, R. E. (1989). *Management* (4th ed.). Englewood Cliffs, NJ: Prentice Hall.

Welkowitz, J., Ewen, R. B., & Cohen, J. (1991). *Introductory statistics for the behavioral sciences* (4th ed.). New York: Harcourt, Brace, Jovanovich Publishers.

Windsor, R. A., Baranowski, T., Clark, N., and Cutter, G. (1984). *Evaluation of health promotion and education programs.* Palo Alto, CA: Mayfield Publishing Company.

Author Index

Subject Index

A

Accounting: A Management Approach, 123
Advance Data, 73
American Journal of Epidemiology, 73
American Journal of Public Welfare, 73
Analytical epidemiology, 73
Arithmetic scale line graph, 81

B

Basic Accounting and Budgeting for Hospitals,
  123
Behavioral Risk Factor Surveillance System
  (BRFSS), 79
Budgeting, health planning methods, 123
  line-item budget, 123–24
    budget justification statement, 133
    clinical materials, 132
    computing office support costs, 127–31
    continuing education, 132–33
    educational materials, 131–32
    miscellaneous costs, 133
    staffing pattern costing, 124–26
    travel cost determination, 126–27
  program budget, 133–34
    example of, 134
  revenue budget, 134–35
Budget justification statement, 133
Bureau of Labor Statistics, 68

C

Case specific rates, 74
Cause specific rates, 74
Centers for Disease Control and Prevention
  (CDC), 68, 73, 79
Closed quantitative interviews, 113
Cluster/area sampling, 105
Community Health Analysis, 73
Computer literacy, 158

Computers, 157–59
Convenience sampling, 105
Critical Success Factors (CSF), 170–71
Crude rates, 74

D

Data analysis, 115
Data collection, document review, 114
Data collection methods, 107
  design, 107–8
    formating/reproducing, 109
    instructions, 109
    item construction guidelines, 109
    item ordering, 109
    question types, 108
    reliability, 109–10
    statements, 108–9
    training, 109
    validity, 110
  interviews, 112–14
    closed quantitative interviews, 113
    informal conversational, 112
    interview guide approach, 112
    standardized open-ended, 112
  questionnaires, 110
    direct administration, 110–11
    mail surveys, 111–12
    telephone surveys, 112
Data reporting, 115–17
Decision support system (DSS), 171–73
Demography, health planning methods, 61–68
  health services utilization, 63–66
  ordering demographic variables, 63–66
    enabling variables: income, residence,
      64–65
    example of, 66, 67
    need variables: perceived, evaluated, 65
    predisposing variables: age, gender, race,
      ethnicity, education, 63